REACH FOR THE
MOON

by

ANDREW ROBINSON.

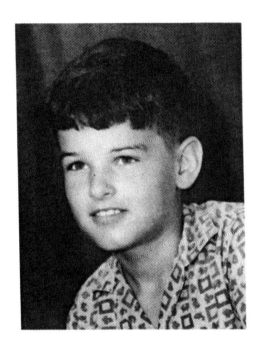

Aged 12

FOREWORD.

My story, which covers five volumes, takes one right through the psychiatric experience.Its roots must lie partly in my past, and in this journey of a soul through the trials and tribulations of an existence more tortured than most I would hope to point out not only the landmarks that signposted my decline but how, when faced with the storm clouds of a major crisis, those embarked upon a similar descent might avert the disasters that the system and individuals who are a product of it can create. I would hope that there are those genuinely interested in change so that where the knowledge and infrastructure exists, with a lock up mentality the trend might be reversed to a philosophy of caring and so give hope to those who succumb to a combination of pressures under which anyone might crumble in the harsh reality of the real world.

CHAPTER 1 (a)
THE NOBLE IMP.

I was born near the end of 1957. My earliest years remain cloaked in the shadows and forgetful darkness that is the nature of infancy with only a few recollections or phantasmagoria illuminating them. These are of Ixopo, a village and centre of a large rural English speaking community in Natal, South Africa where my father was vicar. His parish also included neighbouring villages. The vicarage stands clear in my memory. It was a bungalow with a glass enclosed veranda approached by a long dirt driveway bordering the churchyard.. My mother said that the dead are the best neighbours you can have; they are so quiet. There was a large garden with lawn and plum trees, an orchard with chestnut and tangerine trees and a large vegetable patch growing cabbage, potatoes and rhubarb. Near the kitchen garden were the kiers of corrugated iron where the black maidservant lived. A whitewashed Zulu hut in the garden served as my father's study. In there he had a desk where he wrote his sermons and a roneo machine on which he produced the parish magazine.

My sister was born eighteen months after me, a pretty thing and I was to grow very fond of her.

A single fantasy remains from this time, three or four crones in pointed witches hats stirring brews. The fantasy was rooted in my subconscious as if I expected women (or the ones I came into contact with) to be capable of evil, not that I thought of my mother as such. She did however have a will of her own, she was not truly cut out for or happy in the role of vicar's wife and was inclined to take advantage of my father's philosophy. To force her into a more traditional mould would have required a high handed approach though my father was quite gentle and the notion of him hitting my mother around was inconceivable. I fitted into this cauldron.

We were given some bantams which we kept in a chicken run on the edge of our garden. We fed them everyday on corn scattered over the hard rutted ground. In a separate run we kept some cockerels, a rather angry breed. One afternoon I couldn't resist opening the wire door. I was of a very young age and in relation to me the cockerels were comparatively large. Before I knew what was happening they all started to fly at me. I pelted out of the pen with all four creatures furiously pecking at my heels. I raced past the orchard, round the house, passing some rose bushes the other side. I wailed for my father who emerged with a walking stick and shooed them off.. Back in the safety of the vicarage I declared that such creatures were not fit to live. Joseph, our garden boy, a man aged between thirty five and forty, a friendly Zulu with thick soled feet who used to tramp everywhere in my father's old army officer's uniform, chopped off their heads and we had them for Sunday lunch.

I was often asked to water the vegetable garden standing innocently there in my birthday suit with a hose pipe in hand, spouting an endless torrent of water while the garden boy mowed the lawn, both of us under the discerning eye of my mother who continuously gave the servants orders. My mother was keen on gardening and also liked to get down on her hands and knees to plant seeds and see them grow and sprout out of the rich soil. I never got pocket money though I often got what I asked for, and my reward for watering the garden was a penny.

Though not a belligerent little boy I liked running about and playing. A colonel and his family lived in the house behind us. The two sons were very adventurous and I often went round there as they had an army field caravan, a go-cart and a lovely tree house. I particularly liked the tree house. I was energetic and developing a taste for climbing. As the tree house was so high I was forbidden to go near it. I ventured over one afternoon to discover the family was out. Ambling through the garden I saw my opportunity. I put a foot on the trunk and heaved myself up. The branch supporting the tree house extended quite far. En route I lost my balance and fell to the ground winding myself. I lay there concerned lest I was injured but I was supple boned and nothing was broken.

The country round Ixopo was largely veldt, a crisp dry golden grass that flowed in the breeze. I had a couple of friends whose parents owned two or three general stores supplying the Zulu population in rural areas. We were keen on Noddy and Big Ears. But we liked the countryside and walking more. On one occasion I led them miles through the countryside and though I had a sense of direction I did not of time and we returned late to two sets of very worried parents.

Also my mother bought a mare and an old stallion as the country was ideal for riding, my mother had won a few trophies for riding and was keen on sport especially tennis. But I was never accomplished on horseback.

In Ixopo I was friendly with three sisters who lived on a farm just outside the village with cattle, wattle plantation, arable land and a silo. My mother herself was given an orange farm in Richmond as a present from my grandfather, though he decided to take it back and in addition to wanting to be a fireman or a policeman I wanted to be a farmer.

One thing we liked was to go swimming. We insisted on a paddle and a dip in the high dam, one of two reservoirs on the farm. The girls mother was busy so the maidservant was put in charge of us. We headed off up a steepish farm road bordered on either side by fir trees, until we reached the dam set higher up, collecting water

5

from a small stream. Though most of the time only a trickle was evident the dam had filled to capacity and was wide and deep. I stepped into the shallow end with my sister and two of the friends. We were at an unselfconscious age and unless in the public baths habitually forwent the use of swimming costumes.

What happened at this point no one is certain. Sally, the youngest of the sisters was riding piggy back on the maid near a steep earth bank that formed one side of the dam. It afforded a sharp drop. The maid's feet must have skidded or slipped on the turf underneath her and without being fully aware of the fact they both disappeared. I looked across and saw Sally floating unconscious on the dark brown water. The maid was nowhere to be seen having plummeted like a stone to the bottom of the dam. Clearly there had been a collision of heads. Sally was out cold, and there was no sign of active life. Figuring out what had happened the two other sisters became very distraught and ran for their mother down the dirt track to the farmhouse my sister trailing behind. Unlike the incident with the cockerels I reacted with a degree of aplomb. My mother had taught me how to swim the length of Ixopo swimming pool and how to keep afloat by treading water with my hands. For about five minutes I desperately swam about trying to push Sally closer to the far side of the dam gliding in a gentle slope down to the water's edge. I was only five, it was a difficult operation and it is no wonder I didn't succeed. Fortunately there was the screech of a car and Sally's mother skidded to a halt, throwing off her high-heeled shoes and diving into the murky depths, pulling Sally to the muddy shallows and laying her on to her back on the edge where she gave her the "kiss of life". Sally's lungs had expanded with air and her mother's training as a nurse brought her round. Sally's mother had taken the precaution of making an emergency call. Sally went off to hospital. And a family friend came round and dived repeatedly for the maid. He was not able to locate the unfortunate girl on the dark floor of the dam and her body was only recovered later. At least Sally was alive and she returned from hospital where she had had a checkup smiling and evidently as right as rain.

My father decided to go for a month's leave to England. From a very early age I had a glowing vision of England.. We had a battered old record player in the house, and the only record I had was Christopher Robin, with Teddy Bears Picnic on the other don't know at quite what age I was given it but I would often put it on as a boy and it gave me my first impression of Buckingham palace. When my father returned laden with presents, in particular a set of the Queen's guards, enough for a changing of the guard if not the Trooping of the Colour, I took great pleasure in arranging them on the floor of the morning room.

6

My father often talked about returning to England when he was in South Africa and enquired after several country parishes as if all he ever wanted was to be a country parson in some obscure Devon living.

Stuck right in the middle of the village was the prison, a rather ugly and sinister place with high grey-stoned loopholed walls like a medieval garrison. Every time I passed it would fire my imagination and I once momentarily thought of the prisoners being tortured inside though I instantly corrected any notion of such a thing being right and in fact never believed there was really torture.

The village policeman usually wore a pistol in a holster and to see white policemen armed was something I accepted as normal. Reports that the police flogged young offenders did circulate back to me, though I never met anyone who was actually subject to such a thing in Ixopo and the thought was slightly worrying. I had mixed feelings about the South African police. Having been brought up with a black and white picture of right and wrong I saw them as probably keeping the streets clear of crime whilst I also entertained the contrary picture of them as being rather harsh. The black policemen in their uniforms and pith helmets were often seen peddling along the dusty road near the church on their status symbol bicycles. They only carried truncheons and didn't fill me with any especial fears. My father had brought me up with the notion that the English policeman was humane, the ordinary Bobby on the beat of popular tradition. It was part of the picture handed down by my father of Britain being the mother of justice and centre of civilisation. I was a child and accepted most of what I was told.

One Christmas I was blessed with a bicycle and my sister a tricycle, presents from someone I was inclined to believe in, Father Christmas.

The policeman's son was not so fortunate and while my sister and I were scooting along the dusty road past the entrance to the church, the policeman's son appeared and asked with a hint of envy in his eyes and voice: "Can I have a ride on your bike?" He wore a crew-cut and was a year older than me, a tough little boy, every inch the Afrikaner, reinforcing my father's slightly prejudicial view. I attempted to explain to him that my father had forbidden my sister and I to lend out the two new sparkling pieces of apparatus, but he was very insistent. He resorted to a childish form of bribery offering me one, then two, then three dinky cars in exchange for the privilege. I capitulated and he climbed on and zoomed off stirring up a nice little dust cloud. On returning he got off and clouted both my sister and I on the nose. It must have been quite hard as I vividly remember the sensation of blood trickling down my upper lip. I had been brought up to turn the other cheek and it never occurred to me to hit him back. My nose might have been pushed a little awry.

We reported the matter to my father, that seemed the natural thing to do. He was not very happy and strode angrily to the village policeman's house to voice his disapproval. I remember wondering if the policeman would flog his little boy.

In my heart of hearts, I was, underneath my outdoor exterior, quite a nice little boy. I had some idea of justice and was not malicious quite happily taking to such things as Sunday school. The Sunday school had quite a few swelling its ranks and we would contentedly sit round doing such things as pasting pictures of Jesus and the bible stories into a little booklet we had each been given. For each attendance we were given a new picture to stick in. It was here I gained a foundation in how to live and the bible and I had the picture of Jesus in white Palestinian dress billowing round him, with a beatific expression on his face, encircled by a mass of straight golden hair falling in rich profusion over his shoulders--the paragon of male goodness. I saw God as an old man with a flowing beard seated on his throne on some cloud in the sky. The devil didn't figure much in my thoughts and my idea of him was fudged, the emphasis on such teaching being on the good rather than the bad, and its part to play in life. Not surprisingly I was roped into the embryonic choir one Christmas. It was with an element of pride along with enjoyment of the tune that I embarked upon a solo:

Away in a manger, no crib for a bed,
The little Lord Jesus lay down his sweet head.

The sugar and spice and all things nice mentality was even here gaining ascendancy over the slugs and snails and puppy dogs tails idea of little boys, and a part choir boy mentality was being laid down.

Going to school was an occasion I looked forward to with relish, and I remember putting on my school uniform and cap with enthusiasm, and how I insisted upon a red case for my books. It was just a new adventure for me. As a family we knew the headmaster, as we did the village doctor, and other professional families, my father being the vicar. The headmaster, I knew administered the cane but I only saw his paternal side and it held no terrors for me. I do not recall my father ever laying a hand on me and corporal punishment was very much a new domain. But in the playground I had my first experience of being teased, on this occasion over one of my ears being bigger than the other. At prize giving I discovered I had come second in the form and was given Thomas the tank engine I think as my prize.

Then one day a great big furniture van made its way down our drive, parking in the shaded area between the house and the graveyard. Two overalled men emerged, opened the giant maws at its rear, and gradually emptied the house of all our possessions. I felt quite excited. We were moving to Margate, a new parish on the south coast of Natal, and the prospect of living by the sea filled me with great enthusiasm.

Margate was a growing seaside resort. Sugar cane covered most of the coastline, interspersed with banana plantations. The rectory was built on a slope with three terraces leading down to the whitewashed Anglican church. It enjoyed a fine view of the sea. Across the road from the church was more plantation. Gradually the plantation was being eroded and cut down with increasing development, though there was a resident population of monkeys. You only had to wander a few yards to see them. The beach beyond, marred at one point by the discharge of sewage from a small works buried in the plantation was otherwise very beautiful with rocks and gullies and little salt-water pools where shiny little minnows darted and mussels clustered..

I spent many hours on the beach toasting in the hot summer sun. There was a tidal pool near us where in stormy weather waves used to break. I often went swimming there and the salt and sand clinging to my brown body was natural for me. I tried hard at swimming though only perfected the crawl. I also went to the main beach where there were shark nets.

Margate school was of red brick teaching children to standard five when they went off to Port Shepstone High school. I settled easily into the class, making a couple of friends who interestingly ended up as doctors. I came near the top of the form. Apparently I made an impression on a few of the girls. I was a handsome little boy though I thought the whole business of girlfriends ridiculous and my mind was occupied with fishing and cricket.

My father decided upon a nine month exchange visit to Eye, a parish in Herefordshire in England, and so we boarded a liner at Durban docks and set sail for England, the start of a new adventure for me, and one that was to reinforce my rather glorious eight year old vision of the world.

I attended Eye school. Here I settled down easily. In the playground we kicked a football around, my introduction to the game. It was the year of the world cup and football mania took over. When a match with a neighbouring school was organised we all wanted to play. It was an all winds and weather sort of thing though I was oblivious to the icy chill and wet. There was a bespectacled boy in my class, nice and quiet. Standing on the touch line dressed in my football shorts and shirt, I was slightly inconvenienced when the headmaster came up to me, tapped me on the shoulder and said: "Come off at half-time and give him a go." It was not that I objected to him having a go, but that I was fiercely competitive. I disliked any one or anything getting in the way of my great love, football as it was then. I was wrapped up in the match when half-time came and instead of coming off I did one thing I remember with shame. I decided to continue through. I was a forward and compounded this blot on my childhood when having set myself up neatly in front of the opposition goal I misdirected a kick over or wide of the net ending the match in a draw. Fortunately England won the world cup.

In the village there was the old vicarage which dated back to Charles the first and nearby Ludlow castle. The whole area was rich with examples of the past and I was filled with a sense of history. I especially remember a day out to Goodrich castle, another ruin. I recall crossing the fine moat, exploring the ruins inside, climbing up the keep and descending into a dark dank dungeon. It was very easy for my imagination to embellish these bare details with the flavour of battle and pageantry of the past. Richard the Lionheart along with Robin of Sherwood forest were to form the raw stuff of my picture of the medieval way of life.

I began a collection of Ladybird books around this time including ones on Admiral Nelson, and Alexander the Great. Although not basically aggressive, (my mother said I didn't have an ounce of malice), I saw in these characters a combination of the heroic past and idealism, also love of country. I also started a collection of medieval soldiers.

My last day at Eye school was a slightly mournful occasion. I had been very happy there and I hung round seeing everybody leave, chatting to the bespectacled boy. When he finally had to catch his lift I in turn left the school precincts and said goodbye to a part of my life that I both enjoyed and treasured.

THE WELL OF LONELINESS.

In January 1967, at the start of the South African school year, I was sent off to Cordwalles, a well-known South African prep school on the outskirts of Pietermaritzburg, one hundred and fifty miles from Margate. As the school had an Anglican foundation, and my father was a minister in the Anglican church, I was entitled to go for quarter fees. I had looked forward to going to the school and half encouraged it expecting a whole new world of opportunity and adventure. Immediately on my arrival I sensed the coldness and impersonality of the place. I had been placed in a year with boys nearly a year older than me, certainly they had a year's more education which made me feel at a slight disadvantage, though all my life I tended to feel under estimated rather than inferior, whilst feeling uncomfortable having to live up to great expectations. My initial reception was not warming for a boy of nine. In the dormitory several of the older boys dressed in the traditional khaki shorts and shirts circled round me rather menacingly. A boy called Cartwright with a limp caused by an attack of poliomyelitis at birth, started to flick at me with a towel. This stung leaving a red mark on my thigh, and when the matron entered I went up to her and complained. She gave me a look as if to say "You fight your own battles here" and turned and marched out of the room whereupon the boys rounded on me angrily saying that I was not to tell tales at prep school and that it was "sissy." That night the boy who occupied the bed next to mine, a future cricketing star, was blubbering quite openly. After lights out I rested my head on the pillow and felt like crying my eyes out too, but pride stopped me.

The next morning I was woken by the early morning bell sounding at six thirty. On waking and climbing out of bed we washed our faces and wiped the sleep from our eyes in the washroom next door. We dressed and then descended the stairs following the corridor to the quad where we lined up according to houses. There were four houses, Jackson's, Tathams, Butchers and Baines. I was a "Jackson knight". The master on duty read out the notices for the day before ordering us to lead off. We marched off in two parallel lines down a corridor to the dining hall. As a new boy I had to sit at the bottom of the table. The prefect ladled out porridge into bowls which were in turn passed down the table. We had to eat everything put before us. The porridge was usually edible although on one occasion when a horrible gruel was served up I remember a desire to be sick at every mouthful. The second course was an egg on a half slice of toast served by black waiters in white coats. It was my job to stack the plates which were passed down to me in a pile at the end of the table.

After breakfast came bed making, a new experience for me as the black maidservant did it at home, though I quickly got into the rhythm, being careful to iron out the creases and fold and tuck in the corners correctly. After this we filed off to chapel.

The chapel was at the end of the grass quad opposite the headmaster's study, with classrooms at either side. I had to sit in the gallery where I was able to look down upon the assembled school, the choir in the stalls adjacent to the chancel and the headmaster in the priest's chair conducting the service. There was a short service of worship every morning for which attendance was compulsory. During the beginning of term hymn my thoughts turned back to home, and I suffered a terrible nostalgia and loneliness which was to remain the hallmark of my years at prep school. I had thoughts of asking my parents to take me away again, yet as I had encouraged the thought of being here I didn't think I could do such a volte face and out of sheer pride, gritted my teeth and endured the experience for four years.

After chapel we filed off to our classrooms, one stream to the right, one to the left. The new boys underwent a test and I was lucky enough to pass into the A stream rather than the B, the start of a very poor four years.

Lunch was a formal occasion. After grace we sat down to five minutes of Vaughan William's, or some other composer, when we had to maintain a strict silence while the master at the head of the table dealt out the main course.

During the rest period we would lie on our beds with a book from the junior library. The choice of reading varied but though I happily lost myself in a book I was not imprisoned by them. I followed everyone else's choice from Paddington Bear to Reach for the Sky. Douglas Bader was an instant hero with me.

The afternoon was taken up by sport. Wickham and Cartwright taught me to bat right handed in the nets though I was left handed. I like everyone else caught the cricketing bug and getting into a team was top priority taking precedence over everything.

After sport we had showers in piping hot water supervised by the matron whence to supper with such things as Welsh rarebit on toast and as much bread as we wanted to fill up on. During prep, a half hour quiet period, I would hastily do the necessary work. Then to Vespers. There I knelt and prayed for my mother and father, for my sister, Judy the dog, and to get into a school cricket team. I also prayed I would one day marry the perfect English rose and that I would live in a mansion like my grandfather when he was alive. He had inherited a chain of department stores.

It became apparent that my form was an idle form and I was the idlest in it. I was unhappy being so far away from home and was more inclined to daydream than work.

The dormitory window was situated above my bed and looking out I was able to see the road and swimming pool beyond surrounded by wire netting. There was a strict rule that there was no talking or getting out of bed after lights out. I was kneeling on my bed gazing down at the tarmac below attracted by the sound of a cat and a dog or something fighting below. I promptly informed the other boys of what I had seen and Cartwright climbed out of his bed and limped over followed by two or three others. It was entirely innocent but at that point the dormitory door swung open and the light switch was flicked on to reveal the headmaster's wife looking none too happy in the doorway. We were asked what we were doing out of bed and ordered to report to the headmaster's study.

I had never been beaten and as we lined up outside the headmaster's study I was quite buoyant and carefree. Wickham and Cartwright bragged about having been beaten several times taking it as a big joke. I myself had been spanked and thought a beating would be no more serious not perceiving the nervousness beneath the bravaderie.

The headmaster appeared and called the first one in . The door clicked firmly shut behind him. A short while later there were three loud cracks and then the boy emerged ashen-faced. My turn came and I nonchalantly entered.. The headmaster ordered me to bend over the armchair near the door. He produced a yellow strap with some nasty looking thongs and advanced. I was asked to lift up my dressing gown, he took up his position behind me and then the strap descended on my thinly covered backside. As it bit in I didn't know what had hit me. It was like a thunderbolt. Still unprepared for what was happening it came down again. But I was in too much pain to cry out. I prayed for the agony to end. It descended a third time. I was now free to go making a rush for the door the pain burning itself into my memory.

In the light of the changing rooms we paused to examine our injuries. People wore their weals and bruises with pride though this, my first lesson in discipline, had a subduing rather than corrective effect on me. On entering the dormitory I had already made up my mind I would avoid a repetition.

Our English master, a young man with a beard disguising a bad scar on his face, set us an essay to do one English lesson, entitled The Dark. It allowed my imagination full rein and I enthusiastically put pen to paper pouring out all my fantasies about the evil that takes place under the shadow of night, knives glinting in the pale moonlight, the spilling of blood, ghosts of corpses in graveyards "spiralling" their way to heaven. At the end of the lesson I walked

13

up to the desk and presented it to the master saying what a waste of time I thought it was. When the essays were returned he commented at the bottom it was the most imaginative essay he had read of a boy my age and pinned it on the notice board. The others said it had no story line and were quite scathing killing off any further incentive to study.

The cricket match against Durban North was the one all wanted to play in and after the team had been pinned up we all congregated round the notice board to find out if we had been selected. I was disappointed in that I had not even been made scorer. I was a low run scorer but I thought better than some. When the minibus left with the team I shed a tear knowing that their day of fun, fizzy drink and gluttony had been denied me.

There was an outbreak of flu in the school. One boy fell after another till it reached epidemic proportions with the whole sanatorium taken up with the sick. Eventually I too succumbed with a wild headache and a raging temperature and I was placed in a dormitory that had been turned into a sickbay. The sister ceased to be able to cope so it was decided we should be sent home until we had sufficiently recovered. My mother came and drove me back to Margate wrapped in a blanket in the back seat. I was put to bed and thought "How lucky I am." To occupy my time my mother gave me a stamp album. I had a pile of stamps torn off envelopes and I soaked them in a bowl of water till they came off, let them dry and stuck them in the appropriate countries. Philately was a favourite hobby of mine for a long time. My mother extended my period of recuperation by a week or two and I loved every minute of it.

At about this time sex revealed its ugly head.. Our Biology master had described in detail on the blackboard the mating patterns of the locust whereupon one bright spark commented: "Please Sir. Do humans do it the same way?" That was how I first found out the facts of life though I was shocked to think of my parents doing it. Cordwalles was an eye opener for anyone into the facts of life be it primarily from the wrong end. I learned of something called masturbation. I tried it once, my fantasies probably centred on cricket and I gave it up as a bad job. I did believe there was something bad about sex, a residue from my childhood though what I witnessed I accepted. Mutual masturbation was well-known. Not only did I not participate but could see nothing in it and all I felt was curiosity. The attitude was a hypocritical rather than a matter of general disapprobation and news of an exploit would be circulated. It was not a matter of perversion so much as exploration, the more self-confident, adventurous, individuals pursuing avenues that someone like me, a little insecure in this environment, would refrain from. I was in a dormitory for older boys now and one Sunday evening after lights out a more mature boy climbed out of bed and

14

claimed the boy in the bed next to mine. Clearly he saw him as a substitute girl. There was no romance, just basics. I grasped at least the theory of the mechanics of sex though I had an idea it was frowned upon. The other boys in the dormitory got ideas. I had an invitation. When I got out of bed it was clear that things had gone too far even though I did not indulge in any of the aforementioned things. At any event I never knew of anyone from prep school to emerge as a fully fledged homosexual. The prefect put a halt to anything further at this point and homosexuality became a closed book at prep school.

At about this time some of the more senior boys were shown around Fort Napier. It was the local mental asylum and just thinking of the place gave us the creeps. There was something shadowy and strange to us boys about madness due to a fear of the unknown. One of the boys who went on the visit reported having spoken to a woman who thought she was the archangel Gabriel. In her they might have discovered a fraction of what they had set out to find but I also got the feeling they thought the visit a little flat.

My year was auditioned to join the school choir and we all lined up in a pew in the chapel. The choir master handed round type written sheets of Loving Shepherd or some hymn. My turn came to sing and I launched into the first verse with full throttle my wavering voice reaching up to the vaulted ceiling. It never occurred to me I might be able to sing but the choir master was a good judge and I along with two others was chosen to join the choir. Afterwards there was consternation. One boy complained that the only reason I had been selected was that my voice "wavered like an opera singer's." It was said the cricketing star should have been chosen though he had a slight croak. The choices of the boys were based on favourites.

We would often kick about a rugby ball. One day two of us borrowed a ball from the rugby ball shed and started kicking it over the rugby posts. My partner then decided to go indoors asking me to return the ball when I was finished. On my own my mind wandered off and I walked indoors leaving the ball outside where it warped in the wet. The following morning at parade the headmaster asked the school who had borrowed the ball as it had been left out all night and was out of shape. I miserably owned up though I couldn't explain how my mind had wandered off and denied leaving it out. I had only ever told one harmless lie but had been found out and from the age of five when this happened I never told another but denial was unthinking in this case. Fortunately the shop from which the ball was purchased agreed to replace it free of charge and that was the end of the matter.

There was an election for form head. The class thought I was nice and that they would be able to get away with high jinks so voted for me. Although I was not popular because I found it hard to relate to their mentalities on a personal level I understood power perfectly and when someone spoke during a quiet period my assistant and I determined upon beating the culprit with a steel ruler. I just issued the order to my henchman. But before the deed could take place the headmaster and senior master got wind of what was happening. I just said if I remember clearly: "But you beat boys Sir." I was to keep good control.

I was asked to sing a solo at Vespers one evening, "The day thou gavest Lord is over..." I don't quite know which song. It was a joy to kneel there in the sepulchral gloom of the chapel and feel at one with the universe.

The next morning a boy came running up to me as I stood on the polished corridor outside my classroom. "The headmaster wants to see you" he said. A few minutes before a boy had run across the grass quad to the classroom opposite passing in clear view of the headmaster's study with its wide French doors opening directly onto the grass. My heart almost missed a beat and my knees turned to jelly. A summons from the headmaster. It was the thing I dreaded most in the world. I made my wretched way to the door of his study and waited outside in trepidation. I was convinced the finger would be pointed at me and I would receive the cane. My name was called and I miserably entered. The headmaster was seated behind his broad work desk. "It wasn't me who ran across the quad Sir" I stammered desperately. The headmaster's face broadened into a wide smile and he replied that he had just wanted to congratulate me over my solo the previous evening. Any idea of having made a fool of myself was overshadowed by an overwhelming feeling of relief. He could be encouraging too.

Even so I was not a very popular boy amongst my classmates. I was younger and my thinking different. It was now a challenge was made to my manhood. I was prompted into a fight on the grass behind the tennis courts. It was a hot day, the sun blazing down from a lovely blue sky. News of a fight got round like wildfire and most of the school getting wind of it, came out in a giant surge circling round my opponent and me three or four ranks deep. My opponent was a large boy and had ten months growth on me, the rough and ready son of a white farmer. I on the other hand was the soft spoken son of a white priest unused to the rough and tumble associated with schoolboys. My opponent began by grabbing me in a stranglehold and we fell to the ground in a tight embrace. I was well built for my age and we fought and rolled about on the grass for sometime. The applause was about equal. I was not one to give in easily though it was exhausting. We rose and shifted our positions. My opponent, angry over his lack of success, delivered a sharply aimed blow at my face. I was shocked. Hitting someone in the face

16

was unthinkable to me. But when he continued with his battery of swipes and punches and the spectator applause swelled moving almost completely in his favour I was lost for what to do. It was not necessarily a personal attack against me though to see my friends cheering on my opponent threw me. It was like little boys baying for blood, my first insight into the darker side of human beings. The tears welled up. It was like fighting the whole pack instead of one individual. I swung blindly then turned and walked away. A couple of older boys came over and led me away offering reassuring words. The incident compounded my isolation and I was careful not to be drawn into a fight again.

The end of term was always a great occasion and as we packed our suitcases it was like being lifted to a new plane of happiness. At home I got to know a doctor and his family who lived above in a fine modern bungalow with an aquamarine swimming pool and a large double garage where they kept a speedboat. I initially got to know the son though he had a younger sister whom I met on passing. The son and I shared an interest in fishing as with his father. His sister, a Goldilocks type creature, bouncy and pretty, took a fancy to me and we climbed into the front seat of the speedboat, my sister and her brother in the back. My first kiss was delicious. So was the second, third and fourth. I felt guilty. I wanted our relationship kept a secret from my parents. There was still the suggestion that kissing was dirty. I told my new girlfriend not to dare inform her father. The next morning I called round. The family was seated at the breakfast table with cereal bowls and glasses of juice in front of them. The father swung round on his chair and smiled: "I hear you've got a new girlfriend." I felt myself go red. My confidence had been betrayed so I gave up my girlfriend.

The girl living adjacent was very keen on me and her mother embarrassed me by going on about my handsome looks. Sitting next to me on my bed in my room one day looking at my photograph albums the girl asked me for a photograph of myself. I refused.

Then when I was with my father outside the post office in Margate a lady commented: "What a handsome son you've got."

It was sickening but left me with a belief in my own beauty though I gave up girls as "sissy".

I still saw my old friends from Margate school. I visited one at his parents thatched house in Ramsgate. We still played cricket and a mutual friend and I set up some stumps on the lawn. We each took a turn at batting. My turn came. I faced a few balls but then "Howzat" rang out and I was accused of being stumped. I was convinced I hadn't been. There was no umpire and the friend refused to change his mind, I to budge. After some time had elapsed he and the mutual friend decided that the only way to get me to shift would be to taunt me. They were titches compared with me so the moment I made threatening noises they rushed indoors and bolted the front door. My sister, who was present, had joined them. They stared at me out of the window laughing and making ridiculous faces. I was a little annoyed at that point so I picked up a lump of concrete off the ground and committed the only act of vandalism of my childhood lobbing it through the glass. That I hoped would wipe the smile off their faces. I still don't know how else I could have behaved and retained my dignity. We otherwise enjoyed a very good friendship.

Our neighbours on the other side were the bank manager and his family. The younger son and I went to the main beach a lot during the holidays lying on the sand bronzing ourselves in the hot South African sun or immersing ourselves in the warm Indian ocean. We would observe the surfers taking advantage of the high waves and dreamed of owning a surfboard.

We were also both keen on flying and would cycle up to the landing strip at Margate with its single hangar where one or two aircraft were usually parked. We could not afford a flip but my uncle in the Orange Free State also flew taking the family on a trip and it was my ambition to be a pilot.

During the holidays we visited Durban regularly. One day in my grandmother's mansion my sister started to tease me. I could not stand ridicule so I punched her lightly in the hollow of her spine. She was in no way hurt but my father saw what I had done and was very angry. He gave me a hard spanking. But that was the only time I had laid a finger on anyone and I grew up with the idea you were not to hit girls.

After one stay in Durban we were driving towards Port Shepstone when a little black boy saw his father walking down the other side of a straight stretch of road returning from work, and in pure glee at the sight of him the little boy bolted across the road. My mother was at the wheel, he saw her coming and fled like lightening. She swerved the car just connecting his head with the right headlight which shattered though perhaps cushioned the blow. We crashed into a beacon. The little boy hit the grass on the left hand side of the road. To hear him screaming cut me to the quick bringing tears of anguish to my eyes. The Zulu's from some mud huts on the rounded hillside on the other side of the road, came down congregating round, wrapping him in a Zulu blanket. After an agony of waiting a police van finally came and my mother asked the policeman to take the child to hospital. He had been scalped. I hated the sight of blood unlike when I was younger when there was an accident with bodies all over the road and I was annoyed with my mother for shielding my eyes and not letting me look. The van drove off the father cradling the child in the back. Curiously I felt ashamed that I should have let such a thing affect me and when the manager of the hotel where my mother did a part time reception job asked me whether I cried I profusely denied it as if it was a humiliating mark of weakness.

Back at school I got further behind in my studies still preferring to idle and daydream the day away. Then the boy who I had fought behind the tennis courts and I were summoned to the headmaster's study. He was called in first and a minute later exited abashed. I entered. The headmaster seated in his usual place, his glasses propped on the end of his nose, said it might be a good idea to demote me. I understood that was the fate of the other boy. In an idle form as said I had been particularly idle. Not only did I feel humiliated, I felt totally misunderstood. Conveniently a tear formed in my eye and trickled down my cheek. Sympathy was the single remaining weapon at my disposal. I could stay.

I bucked up my ideas after this taking a more active interest in school curricula. I took the role of Czar in the Nosebag. But more importantly in Maths I suddenly excelled. We had a Maths exam which filled me with trepidation but when the paper was handed round I turned it over to discover it had precisely nothing to do with what we had studied in class. The questions involved logic and related to real life, applied mathematics. It was gratifying when the results were pinned up on the board to see that I had come top. Also my interest in history waxed and instead of my mind wandering out of the window it was caught up in the Wolfe adventure. I was fiercely English in my sympathies and vividly remember him leading his army up a narrow cliff path at the dead of night to take Quebec. It was again gratifying to see when the results of the history exam were pinned up that I had come top.

The entrance exam to Michaelhouse was a formality. We had done next to no work but that was enough. I only did as much as was necessary to scrape by.

The school always rehearsed the hymns for the Sunday service and for the school carol service efforts were redoubled. We were singing "While shepherds watched their flocks by night" when I superimposed my own version:

> While shepherds washed their socks by night
> All seated round the tub
> A bar of sunlight soap came down
> And they began to scrub.

> While Shepherds ate their beans by night
> All seated round the pot
> The angel of the Lord came down
> And swiped the bloody lot.

My shrill voice carried over the heads of the others catching the ear of the headmaster standing singing by the priest's chair and enraged he turned in the direction of the choir stalls waving his hands and indicating to the school to stop. An embarrassing hush fell over the assembled school. He then asked who the boy was singing those outrageous words. Mustering up all my courage I said: "Me Sir." I was ordered to go and wait for him outside the chapel till the rehearsal had finished and with a sense of doom marched down the centre aisle before the gaze of the boys and masters.

I waited nervously in the left cloister outside. I was fairly certain this would merit the cane but the prospect of school holidays ahead had emboldened me so there was no gripping terror or quaking of knees. A few minutes later I heard the scuffle of feet, a boy or two emerged and then the headmaster appeared. He was surprisingly gracious and perhaps understanding my dread of the cane let me off with a warning.

We were in our final year. It was the custom for a boy in the class to read one of the lessons during the carol service and preliminary to this we each in turn had to read a couple of verses from a Christmas lesson to decide who should receive the honour. My turn came and I walked up the chancel step, stood in front of the lectern, glanced at the enormous tasselled bible open at the Christmas story and commenced. I was always good at recitation. It was left for the boys to decide. The carol service was attended by both boys and parents. In cassocks, with a ruff and medallion round my neck I stood in my place amongst the other choir boys in the choir stalls. There was always a vibrancy about the occasion and I was lifted to a new plane. We proceeded with the carols and the lessons. I had not been selected to read the lesson though the headmaster had said I was the best. No, I wasn't a popular boy but I was leaving soon and was just happy it was the carol service and my last night at Cordwalles.

In the early hours of the morning when the whole school was fast asleep I found myself being shaken and woke up to discover a classmate in dressing gown and slippers by my bed. He urged me and a couple of others in my year to accompany him downstairs. We joined up with a few others and then were led off to the safety of the cricket pavilion, a convenient assembly point. A student master was the moving force and he, Wickham and Cartwright had collected a pile of carol sheets and candles from the chapel. The master had expected a good reference for when he left but it had not been forthcoming. Wickham had been annoyed that our year had been refused the annual trip to Pietermaritzburg museum which other fifth formers had enjoyed. The master then conducted us up the rose lined driveway leading to the headmaster's house the shadows of night hiding our progress. He lined us up in a semi-circle, carol sheet in one hand, lit candle in the other. He stood before us like a conductor and said that whatever happened we were to carry on singing. With a downward descent of the hand we commenced:

Once in Royal David's city
Stood a lowly cattle shed...

At about the second verse the dark figure of the headmaster revealed itself at the front door. Clearly he was wondering what all this was about. He advanced slowly towards the young master carolling away as if oblivious to his presence. Quite understandably the headmaster with his distinguished record at the school and someone whom I had grown to respect, was fuming and when the young master would not budge he shook the candle from his hand leaving the master to carry on singing without the carol sheet. "Get off to bed" was the ominous rumble, the boys panicked and there was a mad stampede of little feet for the safe haven of the dormitories, candles and carol sheets being shed on the way. I reasoned to myself that the headmaster would not beat us all and in myself remained quite unruffled. I had been guilty of four showers of tears at prep school earning me the contempt of some boys and as far as my progress was concerned had hit an all time low. But I was not fundamentally a coward.

The following morning, after speeches, I climbed into my parents car. As I drove through the school gates for the last time I felt a sharp pang. It was curious I should be sad to leave a place I so disliked.

Michaelhouse was to prove a happier experience. Cartwright, Wickham, Pappas and I had decided upon Baines. Our choice had been despised because it was a modern house but enjoyed comfortable amenities compared with the other houses which formed part of the original red bricked building with its large open quad and network of corridors. I was struck by the chapel with its rose window and roll of honour in the front listing all the old boys from the school killed in the two world wars.

After idling for years it was not surprising my placing should be low. Sport focused very much on the curriculum though I didn't make the top teams either.

Beating was common. We had to keep our cubicles and beds perfectly tidy. A single crease, a coat hangar on the bed, a slipper out of place or on the floor, could earn you a black mark. Ten black marks within a term would earn you three strokes of the cane. One poor boy in the cubicle opposite me was as good as gold but very absent minded and untidy. Every day or two the prefect would come round and award him a black mark. He was caned all too often. I was fractionally slovenly for a while, accumulated ten black marks and had to report to the prefects study up a flight of stairs in the main quad. I nervously knocked on the door, pushed it ajar and peeped inside. The prefects were blowing water through a cane to make it more supple. I was brusquely told to wait outside. Then the head of house bid me enter again and I had to bend over a chair and he exacted the punishment, one, two then three strokes in rapid succession of agonising pain. I was a bit older enabling me to stand up to it better. This was my sole beating.

There were trips to the Drakensburg and I took the opportunity one weekend to climb one of the peaks. But it was painful and exhausting spoiling somewhat the beauty.

One evening in the half hour quiet period after supper when all the Baines "cacks" or new boys were seated in the prep room reading, writing letters, dawdling, a couple started to chat when the head of house, tall and imperious, opened the door and presented himself. "Okay. Whose talking?" he asked with a note of authority in his voice. The two people who had opened their mouths owned up. "There were more than two of you talking." No one else was prepared to admit they were talking when they weren't. It was decided the whole class should write an essay on something like discipline I think. I disapproved of this as did one or two others. Why should we write an essay when we had not been talking? I didn't mind writing essays. I just objected to the principle of writing this one. So a couple of us resolved to talk about the ridiculous martinet system of authority in the house speaking of the "crumby" leadership and petty regulations that marred our lives. We nonchalantly handed in our essays along with the others.

A short while later the other boy and me were summoned by the house master. He called me into the office and the door shut behind me. He did not look very happy though I never witnessed any outbursts of anger. He informed me that the head of house had handed my essay to him and it was being treated as a serious matter. "You're lucky I didn't beat you for it" he said. He then told me to leave and write another essay that would be acceptable. I had made my point and went off and did so.

On the whole though I had settled down well and was shedding the loneliness of my prep school days.

It had been decided that we as a family would be returning to England. On my final morning the idea of smearing the house captain's bed with toothpaste was raised. I was his fag and once I had left there would be nothing he could do about it. The junior dormitory discussed the matter and just about everyone volunteered to hand over a tube of toothpaste. I went into the senior dormitory and gingerly made his bed being careful to squeeze out every last drop of toothpaste without letting the older boys see.

My father arrived and my cronies in the manner of true gentlemen assisted me with my cases to the car. So I said goodbye to Michaelhouse.

Before we set sail for England we looked around A. Ross and Co. in Durban, my grandfather's old firm. The management was Indian and we were treated like Royalty. It was an unhappy moment as they were selling up to OK bazaars. I wandered amongst the high racks of shoes. It was stocking up time for me. I got something of everything including a multi-purpose penknife.

My father's new parish in England was Payhembury in Devon. We had a red bricked vicarage with a laurel hedge surrounded by green fields in which a herd of bullocks bounded about. Five miles away lived my paternal grandfather who was to hold on for a few more years. He had been to Gallipoli in the first world war though got dyssentry whereupon he joined the Gordon Highlanders. He later became a canon in the Church of England.

CHAPTER 1 (c)
A MORAL DILEMMA.

My headmaster at Michaelhouse had suggested I go to Blundells. That was beyond my father's means. (Only one in thirty went to grammar school and the local school had not got anyone in for years. There were no places at the grammar school and anyway I was too old for the eleven plus so I was invited along to the secondary modern school and after a very quick test was told: "You will do very well here.") Finally after paging through several prospectuses we thought of West Buckland. It was principally my choice. It was set in Lorna Doone country with patchwork fields surrounded by Devon hedgerows, a mere stone's throw away from the furze covered expanse of Exmoor. At an interview with the headmaster it was said I could go there on the basis of my Michaelhouse report, not brilliant but adequate and he indicated that if I did well enough I could be given a direct grant putting it within my father's means. It seemed the best bet so at the start of the spring term 1972 I was duly driven up the tree lined driveway parking in front of the greystone building unloading my cases before being shown to the Brereton house junior dormitory. I was struck on my arrival by a slightly different tone from what I had been used at Michaelhouse with some swearing though the boys were a motley crew covering all ranges of size, shape, ability, finesse. The school had endured a rough patch and had been teetering on the edge of bankruptcy for a while but by opening its doors to the occasional common entrance failure to a more famous school, the rare boy expelled from a public school, supplementing a genuine hard core it had not only staved off disaster but pointed itself firmly in the direction of success again so that it was one of the better academies of learning. The boys called me Andrew rather than using my surname and formal barriers were broken down immediately.

As the academic year started in September rather than in January in England I mercifully found myself placed in a form of boys my own age and from the start found myself fitting into the routine of school work without trouble. I did not do brilliantly at science subjects but I fared well in the arts. In French I was a novice and soon ceased to bother as there was too much catching up to do with a teacher too involved with the class as a whole to give me much time. In history we did projects. I chose the third crusade and my history master detected a sparkle of enthusiasm, even an imaginative flare that won him over.

In the afternoon once a week there was cross country running for the senior school.

It was early evening and I was sitting in the dayroom with a copy of Jamaica Inn open on my lap when a boy marched through the communicating door dividing us from the neighbouring dayroom and glancing at me shouted "swat", an insult according to my prep school code. Though not a voracious reader I did enjoy the occasional book but the tone of the boy's voice was enough to make me put books aside. Fortunately the attitude pervading the rest of the school that work was "poofy" did not take over my form and I did not fall into the trap of indolence that characterised my prep school days.

The prefects were fairly liberal with the cane at this time. During prep a boy tapped me on the shoulder to ask me a simple question and I instinctively turned round. The prefect looked up from his books and said: "Talking in prep." I had to report to the prefect on duty. I rose and marched miserably out of the room, down the stairs and into the tarmac quad trying to locate the prefect. In the Courtenay house junior dormitory the prefect made me bend over an iron frame bed. He took up his position then the cane came down, one stroke then two, then three. Afterwards he produced a little exercise book for me to sign agreeing that the beating was fair. I dutifully took hold of the proffered biro and in a very shaky hand signed my name. I bravely received punishment but rarely did I rebel.

During the weekend many of the senior boys and prefects went out and got drunk, a practice not condoned by the school though there was a hint of 19th C. Rugby. At this time cars were permitted though they were later banned and a few were parked in the gravel car park below my dormitory window. Later I was aroused by the skidding and crunching of tyres and the revving of engines. I was surprised when the two dormitory prefects lurched in drunk waking up the dormitory. Getting drunk though common enough, was something I considered a grave sin but I became tolerant.

West Buckland did excel in the combined cadet force. I elected to join the RAF section and developed a deep passion for flying. A platoon of us would go up to Exeter airport where we would have the opportunity to go up in a Chipmunk. I always opted for aerobatics.

My mother had taught me the rudiments of tennis and Jerome, a classmate and I were selected to play for the school. Tennis was one of the few sports I enjoyed and I was doing better all round.

It was now I took my first few tentative steps into the real world when I joined everyone else in that universally practised vice of masturbation. As a fourteen year old I might have seemed a late starter but it was my first proper glimpse of another dimension starting without problems. The fires of lust burned inside me and I daydreamed about young slim painted whores though I felt trapped by circumstance unable to indulge my lust except by auto-eroticism, a unsatisfactory alternative. I often went home at weekends when a sense of guilt caused me to refrain from masturbation but when the holidays came round the compulsive nature of sex revealed itself and I started even then.

I was on the whole a very moral boy and liked to be seen as such. We were sitting a Maths test when an Indian at whose table I was sitting dared to suggest I had cheated. That was nonsense; I was in the A stream progressing comfortably - none of us were in difficulty - and he was one of the last boys I would have chosen to copy especially as my form placing was higher than his. He persisted so after lunch I waited for him in the dayroom. He was one of the first to enter. The issue was important to me. I was not going to have my reputation smeared by an absurd allegation so I went up to him and punched him hard on the nose. He was taken by surprise and afterwards complained I had displaced a nasal implant. That seemed unlikely but he did shut up and this one trivial instance of violence on my part achieved the desired result though violence was still a last resort.

I was doing quite well and my history master expressed a belief I would one day be made headboy. He also decided to make me captain of the under fourteen cricket team. I was still a low run scorer though I did earn the appellation "demon bowler". I recall a match against Grenville college. It was held away and the afternoon was cool and pleasant with a few Grenville fans watching from the cricket pavilion; my team was fielding and I was out in the covers dressed in white flannels standing thinking. A curious notion hit me. "What was I doing there?" and I felt strangely sad. I was still searching though I hadn't articulated fully for what. It was a period of dawning sexual awareness for my age group with talk increasingly about the realm of women and I enjoyed all-round perfectionism; in this respect I was wondering for the first time if I would match up to my ideas of perfection. And glancing in the mirror I would think: "Am I perfect?" My sister, on showing a photograph of me to her class had received the comment: "He should be a pop star."

Nonetheless a slight crumbling of my confidence was manifesting itself. This could only explain a visitation by five members of the fifth form to the third form dayroom. The instigator was a fifth former in my dormitory. I was told to stand up against the wall near the door and then a tall ginger haired boy squared up to me. I was told I was getting too big for my boots. I know I had unintentionally wounded the sensibilities of the Brereton fifth former in prep when I had said to him as he was supervising us that I expected to get four or five grade ones at O.level and he was only to end up with three passes. And with being captain of the under fourteen cricket team it would have required a strong core of self-

26

confidence to pass it off. The ginger haired boy clapped his hands together over my ears then punched me in the stomach a few times. I stood there impassively absorbing the smacks and blows and only when a few tears started to form in my eyes did he stop. It hadn't hurt very much; the blow was to my self-confidence but I nonetheless felt resentful especially as I had felt helpless to retaliate. That was my first introduction to most of those fifth formers and except for a couple of minor incidents when I had my arm twisted behind my back and when I was pushed over a stile into some mud it was the only time I was bullied at school. But I was again made to wonder. I associated the individuals involved with considerable prowess in the sexual field. I also associated them with a nasty streak. The "nice" boys were not normally playboys. It was a paradox I was to spend much of my life trying to resolve.

After the incident I brooded and thought non seriously and fleetingly of hurting the instigator with a pair of compasses. I also thought of beating up the boys when I was bigger and older though a year later I would just have automatically turned the other cheek.

When the exam results were pinned up on the third form dayroom notice board I found that I had redeemed myself after my prep school trough by coming near the top of the form though I was only allowed a maximum mark of thirty three percent for French. And I was given a government scholarship. One boy in my class was an electrical wizard, a couple had been to grammar school and though the latter two didn't shine particularly it reflected the standard. As a form we did earn a reputation as an academic year giving back the school credibility in the field of studies. A few geniuses had passed out of the school but we claimed no intellectual giant.

School trips abroad were routine and I seized the opportunity to go to Austria on the annual skiing holiday. On the aircraft at Cardiff airport I first fell in love. It was with a girl called Allison who, noticing me from a distance, had pointed me out to a friend and come and sat down next to me. She was a slim sixteen year old with dark hair, a near deity. Strapped in my seat ready for take off I felt self-conscious. This centred on a slight irregularity of the left nostril of my nose due to it having been bent and I found myself overpowered to the point that I kept looking out of the port window in a desperate attempt to conceal it. Allison asked me if I would like to play a game of cards. I declined watching instead the delicate movement of her slim fingers with her blue varnished finger nails as she shuffled and handed out the cards over the fixed table in front of us. My thoughts followed her as she descended the aircraft at Nuremberg where we had been diverted. When I went down to the breakfast room in my Tyrolean chalet type hotel the following morning for my frankfurter and coffee I found I had lost my appetite and a memory of the girl swept over me in a wave of desire and longing. But skiing soon began to occupy my mind. I have a photograph of the whole group from school lined up on the snowbound mountainside in anoraks woollen hats and mittens expertly balanced on our skis supporting ourselves with sticks.

At school my interest in sport began to wane fractionally. When it came to rugby my body did not develop as the demands of the game would dictate and though reasonably tall and big for my age I just did not fill out as expected and many of my cronies caught up with me leaving me of a mere average build. But to me build was not a priority. I laid more store on an Adonis type beauty focusing on little details such as the development of a slight penile asymmetry and possibly one or two other imperfections common in people.

At night after lights out in the senior Brereton dormitory the whispering and chat would now be of other peoples limited adventures with the opposite the boys describing in graphic detail their plunge into the world of carnal delight. Penthouses and Mayfair's occasionally found their way into the dormitory and as with other boarding establishments you could in all probability find one stuffed under a mattress. The outward impression though was quite clean if tales of sexual excess would continue to prompt the majority to even greater frustration as they prepared alone for the time when they would become men.

I had an essentially moral plan of the world and rather than encouraging any cruel impulse suppressed it. A boy in the class with big ears deemed a little slow-witted was encouraged by a Wackford Squeers type of individual to jump open-legged over the hard back of a wooden chair cheered on by most of the form. There was no merit in the exercise and the only reason for everyone's enjoyment was the secret hope and anticipation that he would miscalculate in mid-flight and come crashing down crunching his testicles. There was a funny side to it but instead of urging him on I turned round weighed by a sense of guilt that I, like the others, had found it funny though this was the only bullying I ever witnessed and I would not have been amused had he hurt himself.

I put my name down to be confirmed in the Anglican church. It was expected of me coming from a church of England family though even now I felt a grave strain being imposed upon my childhood faith. None of the questions I wanted to ask in confirmation classes were raised and the old idea of God holding sway in his heaven and all being right with the world did not add up with my own experience and observations of life. All round me I found a lot of the old ideas about how the world was structured disintegrating and in trying to come to grips with my own life it appeared that aiming for a saintly life, following certain goals, honouring your father and mother, loving your neighbour, turning

28

the other cheek, being honest, meant that great barriers were being raised leading me to retreat further into myself whereas the young heathen who formed the majority of my acquaintances were breaking out in a different direction and were happier.

I was a fairly gentle and unassuming individual and at my confirmation at Crediton Cathedral I did not see what I was doing as totally meaningless for I still believed in a civilised society and that Christianity offered a moral framework for how the individual and society should conduct itself. Confirmation itself was treated fairly light-heartedly by the boys and as the candidates streamed out of the pew into the aisle to go up and make their vows, there was a hint of amusement over it all. The red robed bishop standing with a benign countenance on the chancel steps waiting to proceed with the laying on of the hands was one of the few to truly radiate holiness.

I was entering the dark night of the soul. Not only had I been struck by doubts, religious and personal (after two years of normality I had encountered problems with masturbation), but I was continuing to search for something, something beyond my humble lot, something to lift me to a new plane of existence and only now was I beginning to articulate my thoughts, views and feelings on this. I speculated on some great romance; love did appear like a type of madness that most people succumbed to at some time, but I saw it as representing the apex of human experience.

As it was I only had one girlfriend. She was fifteen with blonde hair and a slightly bulbous nose. She did not provide me with the answer. I had spoken to her before but it was at a party in the centre of Payhembury held by a teenage girl acquaintance that I got to know her closely. I was standing nervously in the middle of the crowded room drink in hand listening to Gary Glitter discoursing from a stereo system in the corner when my hostess forced a passage through the melee and said the girl wanted to "snog" with me. I ambled over and slumped down in an old leather settee next to her. We turned to one another and kissed holding each other tightly. I could smell her perfume and feel her warmth. I had looked forward to this first kiss expecting to be overwhelmed with desire. It was a sad anti-climax. I felt little other than a welcome sense of acceptance, as if women would receive me as good enough.

The girl was to prove the picture of loyalty and devotion. We were standing in the garden of her house by the driveway. It was evening, still and quiet. She turned to me and said: "I love you." I replied: "Sure." She was now my secret girlfriend, a secret anyway from my parents whom I thought might disapprove. Her announcement took me by surprise and I felt flattered. But I could summon up no spark of genuine love and I hoped her feelings would die when I returned to school. There a received a couple of

29

sickly love letters and thereupon gave up anyone who did not conform to my notion of a possible soulmate.

A couple of school fellows had been inspired to write poetry notably when they fell in love. Although I rarely indulged in poetry I did attempt to enter the mind of as madman scrawling in an exercise book as if about myself a few words about a demon waging a war of attrition, his armies marching through the hemispheres of my brain gnawing away at the supports of my happiness.

I got to know someone in Brereton house called John. He had a wry sense of humour making a giant issue out of a boy who had soiled his underpants. On losing his father through cancer John had lost his moral guiding light leading to his expulsion from a senior public school. He had more experience of the real world than me and was quite worldly wise, the most sexually precocious in my year.

He was very pleasant inviting me to go drinking with him at the Rolle Quay, a canal side pub in the bustling little river port town of Barnstaple. Here I had my first drink for although my father hardly ever touched the stuff we were following naturally in the tradition of West Buckland boys who would go out and get drunk and we sat for two hours imbibing the alcohol fumes enveloping our brains in an opiate trance. Afterwards we staggered out of the pub, across the bridge and reeled in schoolboy fashion up the High street. Bleary eyed we set about the task of picking up a girl. We ended up in Woolworth's trying to chat up a small redhead of about sixteen and her impish little sister. The whole thing was a new experience to me. How did you approach it? I decided to talk about myself and school saying how well I was doing and that I came top in Latin to try and impress them. It was all very embarrassing. John stood a yard or two away, debonair, practised and at ease. He was used to the ins and outs of women and depended on his physical attributes. He was blonde-haired of average height with heavy eyelids and a neat delicate face marred only by a broken nose. Something in his look must have communicated itself to the girls for after they had walked off the young sister turned and ran back down the pavement hinting that the older one wanted to sleep with him. For me it was a loss of face, for John a triumph and we came to the grand conclusion that looks were the key to sexual attraction. That I discovered was to be only half the story.

A certain softness made me open to propositions. I went on a gliding course to RAF Chivenor. The air base was largely empty with only part of it functional. A handful of other cadets and I occupied a Nissen hut with a coal burning stove in the middle and a flue issuing smoke through the roof into the atmosphere. Our commanding officer entered while we idled by our iron beds. He was a friendly lieutenant who acquired the nickname Betty.

That evening I asked perfectly innocently where the showers were and I was shown to a Nissen hut. I was left alone, turned on the hot water and stepped underneath, the steam rising and covering me in a sort of mist. My escort returned and chatted to me through the cubicle opening and I was conscious of being the object of attention. I put it out of my mind.

The hope was that we all do the necessary three solo flights round the airfield necessary to earn our wings that weekend. We started off wheeling one of the gliders out of a hangar and towing it by jeep to the airstrip. The glider was launched by means of a winch at the far end. I was invited by Betty to help with the launch. We sat in a "cab" an array of hand levers in front of us.

After the launch we drove off in the jeep halfway up the airfield. I sat in the front the sun beating down out of a clear blue sky. The adjusting of my shirt button by a foreign hand though clumsy was unexpected, not quite etiquette and I climbed and sat at the back of the jeep waiting concernedly for the glider to complete its flight and sail down to a pleasant landing.

The squadron leader took me up. Again I loved the freedom and the quiet as I looked down upon the boats washed upon the estuary sands. I was asked to land the craft nose-diving then abruptly trying to level out. We hit the turf with a few bounces. The squadron leader's heart must have missed a few beats as he seized control of the joystick. I was only conscious of fear when I thought about it.

Betty thought there was not enough time for me to qualify that weekend. He wanted me to return the following weekend. I was a restrained individual with a natural inbuilt block to experimentation. I was agreeable when the squadron leader interjected with an opposing view and I completed the requisite number of flights.

It was time for us to start thinking of a career. It had been suggested I try for the RAF as a pilot , the typical schoolboy dream which for a long time I had been trying to bring to fruition. My Godfather had been in the Royal Navy and I considered that. In the end I elected to try for the Merchant Navy. I paged through several careers books and thought of being a navigating officer. It required the eyesight of a hawk and two of us went by train to Plymouth for an eyesight test. My turn came to read the letters but close work had engendered mild myopia, I couldn't read the bottom lines, and my ambitions to join the navy or be a pilot were dashed in one fell swoop. Afterwards we looked round Debenhams where the "friend" ordered a lounge suite then complained that the colour was wrong when it came to paying for it. We bought a bottle or two of wine and on the train journey to back Exeter he went round asking the passengers to sample it and express an opinion. He was a close friend of John's and joked a lot about their favourite joke, that of sawing off peoples arms and legs. We stopped at Exeter where we went to a disco. On the steps a large crowd of young people had gathered. Strangely a girl singling me out tried to wound me so we left. At the vicarage a couple of girls turned up on the doorstep one day asking to see me. I hated being gazed on. Praise was a form of criticism and criticism could be good or bad. We bought a pint of beer in a pub and settled down at a table where a woman with a red dress was sitting. We bemoaned the frustrations and miseries of a monastic existence such as we enjoyed at school. She was thoroughly sympathetic. We left to arrive back a few hours late and I went and got a hideous pair of National Health spectacles for pick up and put down wear. Some counsel said that they and a teenage outbreak of spots were the two things marring my appearance.

O.levels came upon us. I had prepared quite well for them. With top grades in a couple of the language subjects I thought I would concentrate on them in the sixth form. And I discussed taking up French with the head of the French department in the headmaster's dining room. Although I had made excuses why I should seek employment rather than enter the sixth form, with the toppling of my two career ambitions all objections to my entering the sixth form had been removed. I had spent three weeks in Anglet with a French boy on an exchange visit when I had picked up the accent and a useful store of words on which I could build. I insisted on doing French A.level even though it meant starting virtually from scratch. The two other members of the tutorial sat patiently while the head of the French department staring down his aquiline nose at me tried to dissuade me. He expected the whole class to get top grades which for a beginner would be hard, and it was a difficult A.level. I won in the end. I also elected to do Economics and English.

Mark Watts and I decided to share a study in the sixth form study complex. Mark had come from a broken home and was amoral and worldly wise distinguishable by his thin delicate bone structure and light fuzzy hair. He aspired to be an aesthete and seated in our study would spout extempore poetry. We started by both giving up the CCF though I had my marksman's badge, I had passed an exam in the principles of flight and had been told I could expect to lead the platoon and earn my sergeant's stripes. The ultimate function of the military man appeared to be to kill people and though as a boy I had enjoyed it when I went hunting with my uncle in the Orange Free State following the trail of blood left by a "dussie" he had shot, killing was now anathema to me as it was to Mark. We also refrained from sport and rugby which we argued demanded a Neanderthal approach to life. I joked that in the event of a war I would be a conscientious objector on the grounds of cowardice. Instead of destruction we were preoccupied with creativity and beauty became our ideal.

Sometime that term I did a career's test for sixth formers round the country. Although I did not do as well as I could have had I been in gear which I wasn't because of my moral passivity, I did score university entrance for the Arts. Linguistic ability and creativity, my strengths were not assessed and the tests could not be taken remotely seriously.

I went on the annual skiing trip to Austria in the Tyrol sharing a room with a balcony in the hotel. We headed for the bar downstairs perching on stools swigging Schnapps. In a bleary haze we then stepped into the crisp cold Austrian evening skidding and skating down the frozen iron hard road. Coming in our direction were the products of a girls school staying in a hotel down the road. I was struck by a creature in a red anorak with lovely blonde hair, the most exquisite button of a nose and big blue eyes. I made a fool of myself with her I was so awkward though she saw in John who was hovering nearby someone more experienced in the ways of the world walking side by side with him. But though my hits greatly outnumbered my brush-offs (aforementioned), to sense the object of my desire slip so easily through my fingers was humiliating.

Later out on the balcony I cursed my lot in life. Romance, joy and fulfilment came so easily to others. To me love was an elusive dream thought about rather than sought as a rule. Tears of frustration sprang up in my eyes.

A little later I was irritated to see a friend of mine dancing up and down with glee having been going on to the girls as if I had never had a girlfriend, nonsense, though I was perfectionist without much opportunity of fulfilling my ideals and I seized him by the lapels. He had no understanding of the weight of repression I endured.

Flea, a tough wiry individual made a bee line for Theresa and his nineteen years reflected a wealth of experience. The two were sitting side by side in the dining room at the end of which the bar was located and I came up to her and said: "Is he what you call good looking?"

It was always necessary to get the feel of skis again and I started again pottering about the nursery slopes, the pine-covered snowclad mountain lowering over us, tall, majestic and overpowering. In the distance the small figure of Theresa gliding over the snowflats was discernible and though my heart reached out to her I let her go in the direction she chose. And soon my mind was concentrated on the majesty of the Alps and the beautiful Tyrolean landscape stretching to Innsbruck, the old medieval city which after a few days of skiing down mountain sides we would visit.

On my our last night standing outside Theresa's balcony John prompted me to shout out that she should enter the Miss World contest. She replied that I was sweet and back at school I wrote a poem in her honour.

My passive outlook and inevitable limited retreat into myself was now leading to a certain amount of self consciousness and this any slight rebuff would accentuate. There were a couple in the form who started to go on about my looks in a disparaging way though I was better looking than them; they were just taking advantage of my doubts. I was hypercritical about looks though the difference between me and other boys was that whilst they condemned others I condemned myself.

John and I were junior dormitory prefects. We kept adequate order though it was my view that the boys do what they want within reason. John's prowess as a lover was becoming legion and details of his exploits were spreading through the school. I scrutinised his appearance but though there was something girlish in it, gender differences came between me and any sexual attraction. I did however have a wayward thought in line with the enlightened male: "Would it be possible to convert myself to a homosexual way of thinking?" These barriers that had been raised between me and men were nothing more than prejudice. I myself was never to foster nor indeed experience a proper emotion for a male, the true indicator of homosexual bent.

I was asked to be house captain. But the summer holidays before the upper sixth when I was to take up the position I went on another trip to France with a group of young people. My mother thought the world of me still and I was very much the person she wanted me to be, occasionally sticking my head out of my shell to survey the horizon but usually leading an inner rather inoffensive life avoiding doing what my generation was doing, going out there, living it up and enjoying itself.

At Thonon-les-Bains I shared a room at the top of a high rise block of flats. Our hosts were very friendly and at the meal table we would be expected to top our glasses with vin ordinaire, stuff ourselves with croissants and be merry. Wine women and song was their motto. They took us to a traditional French wedding which was the highlight of the holiday. The fifty strong group on the holiday attended the lycee for an hour or two each day and we were given a project to do. I described a French wedding in French and won. I recall returning late one night to discover my hosts and some of their friends sipping whisky in the dining room. I was invited in and offered a glass. A transparent dildo was produced filled with milk, the host applied his mouth to the root and after a lot of twirling and manipulation started to shoot milk in sharp vigorous spurts across the table. Although I was to correspond with a French and an Irish girl later my tendency was to withdraw. I was perhaps a little unsure of myself. And in the shower after a swim in Lake Geneva I examined myself. As I looked down, to my horror, I discovered one testicle hung lower than the other. "Have I ripped myself?" I thought. Back at school I started off my time as head of house rather unceremoniously asking Jerome, a soft mannered though inwardly strong crony of mine, what I should do. He replied with typical self-aplomb: "Oh, nine out of ten men are like that."

My father was anxious for me to go to Oxford like he and my grandfather had done. It was supposed to be a practice run as I had not even completed the A.level syllabus and it was unrealistic to think of passing an A.level let alone entering this great academy of learning. I chose English, a particularly competitive subject. Worse my brain went on strike when I sat the entrance paper so I only wrote half a page. But I was called for an interview. Hardly anyone went to Oxford from West Buckland. It geared people for the provincial universities which was where I expected and wanted to go. In the hall of residence that evening I sat amongst a collection of literary geniuses and listened to them spout in golden tongues on all aspects of Oxford life. They reminded me of BBC presenters. Apparently there were women at Oxford. The scholar was said to have worn out several pairs of shoes tramping to a woman's academy of learning on the outskirts. The streets of Oxford were supposed to be busy with the odd student being carried away on the bonnet of a motor car. I was intimidated by their pyrotechnic display of brilliance. The next day I was nervous about my interview and when asked from the study above the beautiful old quadrangle of Worcester college why I had written so little I said the quotations in the English paper which we had to expand into Francis Bacon type essays had unarmed me. Quite rightly Oxford felt it could rub along without me. I was relieved rather than disappointed and had no intention of resitting the Oxford entrance. I was more conscious of my burgeoning sexuality rather than interested in academic plaudits. But my companion on the trip got a place to read Chemistry at Brasenose.

The school treated me more kindly and on speech day I had to walk up on stage first to collect the house cup in my capacity as house captain of the winning house, then the Shepherd Law scholarship for the best O.level results, then the verse speaking prize and English prize.(This was due to having the best teacher I had known.) Afterwards I was photographed with some dignitaries clutching the house cup. But still I did not aspire to be an egghead preferring the idea of being a quiet pin up settled in connubial bliss, my emotional and psychological needs in happy equilibrium. But I was in no-mans land emotionally and physically sexless.

The sixth form dance was the highlight of the term and there I met Beverly. She had noticed me before having gone out with another boy. But the ingredients making up the chemistry between us were not correctly mixed and three weeks later in a pub in Biddaford where some sixth formers were gathered I suggested she go to a disco with some others. She insisted on waiting for me though in the disco she then wisely went off with her former boyfriend. Her tiny wisp of a frame and blond curly hair appealed to John who later went out with her.

I was more absorbed with school activities. Mark Watts had been elected chairman of the Phoenix society and at its first debate in the Geography room chaired by Mark smartly attired in bow tie and jacket I was chosen to defend the motion that The Monarchy Should Be Abolished. I rose from my place and though my instincts opposed the idea I spoke of democracy, the western ideal, and the contradiction between that and a hereditary monarchy. I also spoke of privilege and the social injustice of the monarchy's wealth compared with the relative poverty of the average man on the street. My opponent replied that the monarchy was part of our heritage. The vote was taken. Only a few hands rose for the motion. A host of hands rose against it. The sixth form had voted according to instinct though the French mistress, who was present, did say I had won on arguments.

I was president of the sixth form society organising films for the sixth form. I also edited a magazine called the Blueprint for which there were satirical and political contributions and though there was only one edition it was a success, not so my part in the school play, The Man Who Came To Dinner.

I plodded on alone but if I had used my sense and gone out with women gathering knowledge and experience and understanding rather than just waiting for the one great romance that would change my life, I might have got on perfectly adequately. I think of a dance held at a nearby girls school during my final term to which the sixth form was invited. Present at the dance was a silky-haired girl, regular featured rather than beautiful but with a warm intelligence which had appealed to me on two other occasions I had met her. She was also advanced in her sexual education. After a dance or two we left the dance hall stepping out into the fresh summer evening wandering across a finely manicured lawn towards some balustraded steps leading up an embankment. She sat down on the middle step, I on a lower one. We could hear the music wafting from the dance hall but otherwise it was perfectly peaceful. She said: "You've got a beautiful body." I started stroking her foot moving my hand slowly up to her calf. She slid her frock up over her thighs revealing two long slimly proportioned legs glistening like ivory in the evening twilight. I was curious rather than lustful. But only at the end of the dance did I advance my hand further than the knee when it was too late. The girl did ask me to meet her at a pub the following weekend. I thought it a prime opportunity to lose my virginity.I had always thought of losing your virginity as a great event, as crossing a new frontier in human experience, the frontier dividing boyhood from manhood. But though I found her attractive I was too frightened of failure to consider turning up.

After that things began speeding towards some sort of a finale and into this saga John had inevitably been drawn. Although I did respect his power over women he did possess many base qualities which I loathed and despised because they flew in the face of everything I had been brought up to believe in and I did not fully understand that the delight he took in putting people down and being loathsome was an element in his success in the same way that I did not appreciate my own attempts to fit in with my parents and to accord with my own father's notion of being good or "nice" was a major obstacle towards my becoming a grand seducer and conqueror of women. I believed a harmonious and successful union to be an ideal and John took a gloating satisfaction in my descriptions of the gap between my life as I felt it was and how I would like it to be. Our friendship might have been close but though I spoke to him as if he was a paragon and though I practised my mock brand of hero worship there was no genuine deep emotional or physical understanding outside friendship. And all too soon I began to sense that rather than being my friend and ally he had set himself upon some pedestal and was looking down at me.

One evening I came back from a bout of carousing in a pub in South Molten and I was reasonably tipsy on cider. I marched into John's study and slumped down in a faded old armchair. I was feeling a bit fed up and a bit low. John was someone I believed I could do without and I decided that the best way to bring an end to matters would be to shock him. But as I had suppressed any hint of nastiness or aggression in my personality my approach naturally tended towards self-destructiveness. John's study was dimly lit which I saw would serve to disguise the reaction on his face as well as being quiet and private. He was seated in a hardbacked chair by his desk. Hiding my face with my scarf I proceeded to explain that our friendship had become too involved for the good of either of us. Greek love was almost indiscernible at West Buckland though I was influenced by writers I read, usually modern, and in trying to emulate them I could not exclude all male love. Although I might like love to have existed or to pretend it existed in my life I was devoid of it. But in my idee fixe for beauty I included John in my plan and probably gave him the suggestion of an Oscar Wilde, Lord Alfred Douglas type friendship. In reality it was Wilde's image as an aesthete that appealed to me, not his sexual proclivity. I threw John's mind into a state of confusion, the damage had been done, and after concluding that we should have nothing more to do with one another I rose and walked out of the door.

I was not openly conscious of exam pressure but A.levels were not far off and there was a tension in the air. Two or three of Arabic and Indian ancestry now adopted the curious routine of revising at three o'clock in the morning. They were "quite a laugh" and I didn't take action or report them but it continued. After being woken up for a third time I high spiritedly picked up a slipper from by my bed and threw it hitting the dormitory window with a splintering and shimmering of flying glass.

I was not actually annoyed then but my feelings towards John were not quite so amenable. He was pursuing me all over the place no doubt because I had put him in Coventry and he was unused to it. When he located me he would try and debase me. I spent a fair amount of time in my study in the new sixth form block trying to revise or catch up. Having only taken up French in the sixth form I had to work hard the first year eventually running out of steam and I had a couple of Moliere plays to read. After being called a degenerate by my Economics master for acting as if I was going to sleep in his class I had a little catching up to do there which I did one week in the holidays putting me near the front of the class so I didn't have any worries there. He unsaid his initial comment in consequence adding I was a good prefect. But in English I had neglected a couple of set books feeling they bore no relevance to my own life. John didn't help barging into the study breaking wind or making rude remarks.

One weekend John came up to me in the sixth form common room and asked me to go drinking with him. A Friday or Saturday evening was the time for letting off steam and a few other members of the sixth form had gone off carousing. John had asked me to go out with him on a couple of occasions subsequent to our rift but I always declined for I continued to see him as a pest rather than a true friend. He just wanted company for the journey which would otherwise have been tedious and time consuming. After much persuasion he succeeded and we set off for the market town of South Molten. We walked steadily skirting a wooded valley and some pasture land in the direction of the main road. On reaching it we were already both hot and sweaty and would have appreciated a lift. We stuck our thumbs out but none of the passing cars stopped and by the time we reached our destination we were both thirsty and tired making straight for a cider den commonly frequented by boys from West Buckland. We must have miscalculated for none of our cronies were evident. Perhaps they had gone to Barnstaple? After a pint John ambled out in search of familiar faces. He didn't return and after consuming a second pint of cider I began to feel a little put out as if I had been brought there on false pretences. I went off and had a third pint in another pub speculating that he must have gone to track down an old girlfriend.

On returning to school later that evening after another long and exhausting walk of six miles I entered the sixth form block where I discovered John looking very pleased with himself. After the recent accumulation of little humiliations capped by the events of the evening I didn't feel too happy. With a fierce mien I approached him. He fled to the sanctuary of the common room retreating into the back of a red vinyl chair where amongst the other sixth formers he felt safe. I came up and tried to provoke him to some stand. He fled to his study bolting the door. I didn't mean to look so serious. I myself professed cowardice but was kind. John it seemed had a yellow streak. I spoke to an Indian friend in his study. He produced a little maxim for me from a used Christmas cracker: "Friendship is like a vase. Once it has been broken it can be stuck together again but the cracks will always show." The incident, though not too serious was to turn John with ultimately tragic results for me.

With June rapidly approaching we had started upon a fairly hectic programme of revision; in my case it was a last minute attempt to catch up. I was supervising the fifth form for prep one evening seated at the head of one of the tables in the conservatory. There was a boy chatting and making a nuisance of himself in prep. I told him to keep quiet. He didn't so I sent him out of the room. He knocked on the door begging to come in again in case the master on duty appeared meaning he might be caned. I let him in again and he promptly started talking again. I went downstairs to Mark's study and spoke to him. He considered beating the boy with an umbrella stick but agreed it should be a matter for the headmaster. So I sent the boy to the headmaster. I felt I had work to get out of the way and that meant I had to be more strict. By his reaction afterwards I can only assume he got six, the only person I had punished during my time as a prefect; my view was that the cane, which I had experienced on three occasions, was barbaric. Although I managed to get a little revision done and walked into the examination room fairly nonchalantly the examiners were too hard that year with only Mark and I passing the English paper. It was pleasant to go home and escape the regimentation of school. John passed out of my mind the first day. But of school I had learned nothing of real life and little did I know that the outside world was waiting for me just like a shark with its jaws wide open.

CHAPTER 2
IN SEARCH OF PERFECTION.

One cold damp afternoon in the September of 1976, after a long drive up from Devon, my father dropped me off at Lancaster University. Most of the boys in my year at school ended up at university though for me it was a last minute decision. Lancaster University was a vast shiny modern academy of learning with some four thousand students, a veritable hive of young life, and as soon as I entered the Fylde college lobby I was swamped with students proffering me literature on the various clubs and organisations and I quickly found myself plunged into the social whirl. People who like me, have spent ten years in the private school system, often take five years to catch up though usually try to do so in three months and though I was supposed to be studying Economics I straightaway became preoccupied with studying life.

In that respect I started with an unexpected success and romance which had so far eluded me now it seemed had its chance to flower. Indeed I found myself the subject of considerable admiration and as I walked down the spine of the university the prettiest girls in the university smiled at me. Whilst I didn't mind this from a distance when they started trying to approach me I became awkward and self-conscious. Again the prime consideration was to prevent a closer inspection whereby a fault might be revealed shattering any possible illusion of an infallible Byronic charm still indicated by a view from the distance. An unexpected consequence of this was the more I avoided or ignored them the more they pursued me.

On my floor in my hall of residence in Fylde college there were six of us. Most were from working class backgrounds but were enlightened and politically conscious and in the self-catering kitchen one day we sat round discussing the Rhodesian crisis with them backing the terrorists and I the Smith regime. We also went drinking in the university and the medieval town of Lancaster and in addition to picking up certain socialist ideas with a strong moral core we had fun.

Despite my initial nervousness over the female half of the campus, I could have made inroads. I think of a girl in my English seminar - English and Maths were subsidiary subjects of mine - who showed an interest in me. She was of slim build with straight brown hair and fine features, warmhearted and delicate rather than beautiful. Our set books in English included King Lear and being keen on English and Shakespeare I always had a ready answer should the tutor fire a question at us. That was the first thing that drew her to me and after a voluntary drama session in the university theatre when she took the part of Cordelia and I the old King Lear she invited me over to her room for coffee. Through shyness I made some excuse not to go.

In my hall of residence there was one good looking girl with many ardent admirers. One evening I rolled up at the first floor kitchen twirling an umbrella. I was feeling a little drunk and carefree having just come from a cheese and wine party put on by the literary society. This girl and a friend happened to be in the kitchen and I asked if I could borrow some butter. I then asked jokingly for some bread and then a toaster or something. For a moment I had totally forgotten myself meaning I was no longer awkward. The awkwardness had probably been more disfiguring than any physical imperfection. Everything I asked for was refused but we got talking and I was projecting myself in a way I hadn't done for years. We discovered a common interest in T.S. Eliot and discussed Murder In The Cathedral by T.S. Eliot then I did another twirl with my umbrella and left. I was a little disconcerted and worried to be followed by several peals of girlish laughter as I descended the stairs. But the girls always gave me a smile and went out of their way to try and talk to me. Early one morning the pretty one even decided to turn up at my door in her nightie and dressing gown whilst I lay in bed on the pretext of wanting to borrow a book. But certain niggling doubts remained. Was I an equal?

It was a natural progression that I should have the fault to my nose corrected and so recover not only the untouched lustre I had enjoyed as a boy, but my boyhood confidence. I did believe there were people around with the skill to do that and really my fault was so petty I could not envisage any problems. I discovered that all that was really required was a straightening of the nasal septum which had been bent either through natural causes or because of the punch on the nose I had received as a toddler. With my looks complete I could happily go on to win the perfect woman and achieve that zenith, a fulfilled love. Three weeks into my first term at Lancaster I sat down at my built-in desk and set about writing two letters to cosmetic clinics whose addresses I had gleaned from the Sun and from an advertisement in the Lady. In my letters I asked three basic questions. How much does the operation cost? What is the success rate? What is the appropriateness of a man undergoing it? But though after posting the letters I attended lectures and socialised as usual I did wrestle deep down with these problems. I thought that by skimping and saving I might be able to afford the treatment. I recalled two boys at school who had had broken noses fixed and the results had been worthwhile. If they had had such a thing why shouldn't I?

On the third day I went up to my pigeon hole in the mail room and there I discovered two letters. I guessed that they were from the clinics. I hurried back to my room and having carefully

41

closed the door I opened them in turn. The first was from the clinic whose address I had found in the Sun and it said that it had a long waiting list. The cost of the correction would be £400. The second letter sounded more hopeful. The cost of the correction would only be £300 and there did not appear to be a waiting list.

After reading the letters I went on to write to my parents on the subject. If anybody had anything to say that might dissuade me from the idea it was them. Three days later I received a reply from my father who said that the family couldn't see anything wrong with my nose and that they didn't want the existing one damaged. Obviously I hadn't made it clear that I was in pursuit of the ultimate and I was not swayed.

That same morning I telephoned Dr.H., the cosmetic surgeon at the second clinic, and arranged for an interview. Dr.H. spoke with a German sibilance, I assumed that he was a German Jew, and he sounded very encouraging. He agreed to see me in the afternoon two days later. As I was telephoning I noticed a very attractive young female student smiling at me admiringly from the distance. "Christ, what an irony" I thought.

I made a telephone call to Mark Watts. He was now living in London and as the interview was to be held there I thought it would be convenient to stay with him. Though I never revealed to him my worst failings I found him very useful as an advisor in the affairs of the world and thought he could counsel me. It was agreed I spend a night at his flat.

The date of my appointment arrived. I caught the university bus to Lancaster and boarded a train for the first leg of my journey to London. On the journey I began to read War and Peace. I was excited but not so excited as to be unable to read. I was convinced that going to London was the right thing. I took it all as if I was going to see a doctor about having my tonsils out. It all seemed elementary, the interview then the operation then the world.

At Euston station I bought an underground ticket to W1 where my appointment was to be and arrived there half an hour early. I wandered around Selfridges for a bit then made my way to the clinic. I pressed the buzzer and an auburn haired nurse answered the door.

The clinic had once been a comfortable residence and had a cosy feeling. In the waiting room there were a couple of armchairs, a mirror or two and a table on which rested a pile of magazines. On closer inspection these turned out to be the Countryman. The nurse left and I picked up a copy, sat down in one of the armchairs and began to browse through it.

The nurse came in again and asked me upstairs. The room upstairs was very plush and had a couple of armchairs, a wall mirror and wide curtained windows. It also had an alcove in which there was an operating table and a cupboard on the wall containing instruments.

Dr. H. appeared. He was a short middle-aged man with a very wide face. I guessed that at some stage he must have had a rhinoplasty giving him that unfortunate appearance. "Christ I don't want to end like that" I thought. But he seemed very friendly. He asked me to stand still and in the presence of the nurse walked round doing a reconnaissance of my back, front and profile. He quickly identified the fault that had concerned me, that of the left profile.

"Does it worry you?" he asked.

"Yes."

At last I felt that someone really understood. Not only was he not afraid to attest to an imperfection but he offered a cure. I imagined that my future was mapped out for me now. Dr. H. stood me in front of the wall mirror and referring to my nose said:

"Perhaps you would like it smaller?"

I thought that it looked just the right size but small noses were considered handsome and I was at the stage when I believed the expert always knew best. I didn't try and disagree with him. He asked me to lie down on the table in the alcove, pushed up the tip of my nose and looked down my nasal passages. A bright light was shining overhead to help in the examination. When I was on my feet again he asked:

"When would you like it done?"

"As soon as possible" I replied. "But I'll have to get hold of the money from my parents."

It was the first time I had thought of asking them for assistance. The nurse led me downstairs to a third room. She asked me to sit down in a chair, produced a polaroid camera and took a picture of my left profile. It was by far the most unflattering photograph I had ever seen of myself and though it exaggerated the size of the nose it did serve to convince me that I was doing the right thing. After I had been shown the photograph the nurse asked me for £5, the cost of the interview, with the words:

"I know it's hard."

After paying up I left for Mark's dwelling. He lived in a flat in South Kensington with an old lady. He was not welcome at home so had to fall back on his own resources and though I felt on my arrival that the flat was rather drab it was fairly comfortable. I was given the boxroom to sleep in. After I had been introduced to the old lady, Mark and I sought the privacy of his own room where he asked:

"Why do you want your nose done?"

I replied that I wanted to look perfect.

"But it's a complete waste of money."

43

"On the contrary, I think it's a very sound investment. It will stop me from being awkward. It will give me increased self-confidence. It will help me to relate better to people. £300 is not a lot to pay for that."

"Well, as far a I can see you are just totally selfish" he replied.

"It will make me a happier person. I don't see that that is necessarily selfish."

"Quite frankly I wouldn't mind looking like you. You won't stop at the nose. You'll go and have everything else done as well."

"It's only the nose that I am concerned about."

Clearly Mark did not understand my objections to the nose properly but he did concede there was a little room for improvement. I asked him if I could borrow his telephone and he agreed. I dialled through to my parents in Devon. I spoke to my father asking him if I could borrow the money to have my nose corrected. He was still unhappy about the idea. My mother came on the line and asked me to wait till I was twenty five. I heard her tell my father that on no account should he lend me the money. I handed the phone to Mark who spoke to my sister.

"It's utterly absurd" he exclaimed.

"Can't you dissuade him" said my sister.

It seemed that the only person who understood was Dr. H. though he had a vested financial interest in the matter. It was agreed that the matter be postponed till the Christmas holidays.

When I left Mark's flat the next day I made my way to Euston station and boarded a train for the North full of hopes. I managed to read a few more pages of War and Peace but even then my mind was more on my nose than my book.

But after I had got over the initial euphoria of seeing Dr. H. certain doubts set in and back at Lancaster University I began to reflect more deeply on the wisdom of what I was doing. My doubts began almost to plague me over the next few days but they were not enough to make me change my mind. My major doubt was whether Dr. H. was right in his plan to make my nose smaller as it looked just the right size and I didn't want to go radically changing nature. I just wanted a simple and very minor correction. I thought that with a change of identity it might even be unwise to return to university.

A month before the end of term I stopped attending Maths lectures and ceased to take my studies seriously. Had I truly believed I would attain what I wanted I would not have been worried. As there seemed no point in study I was left but to see what else university had to offer. The first thing was friendship and I spent much time with the male students on my floor in my hall of residence staying up till four in the morning singing along with the

Sex Pistols, I Am An Antichrist. I also got drunk far more often. Although I socialised I did not have the desire to socialise and avoided associating with the second sex except on a superficial level. Whatever the high jinks it was not the happiest time of my life.

Two weeks from the end of term there was a party in the college. This provided me with new opportunities because I decided to go in disguise which meant I could be myself without worrying about my appearance. Being in fancy dress so to speak could give an indication of how I would function without inhibitions. I made two slits for my eyes in a brown paper bag as well as a slit for my mouth and placed it over my head. I drank two or three pints of cider in my room just to get into the party mood. The party proved heaven. My true personality did express itself and I approached at least three of the university belles with the aplomb and charm of an accomplished roue. I was warmly received and knew that as a complete person I would be accepted.

On the last Saturday before the end of term I went to Morecambe with a fellow student by bus. We had a pint of beer in one of the pubs on the seafront. Then we walked along the promenade. It was a calm but cold day and there were seagulls circling and wheeling overhead. I felt a great sense of freedom, a oneness with nature. The promenade ended and we started to walk over bare rocks interspersed with grass. We came a cross a little Norman church tilting towards the sea. It was a fascinating relic of the past, a mark of simple faith, a symbol of man's hope for the future. I was greatly moved. On the walk to the bus stop I encountered a beautiful female student coming in the opposite direction. I saw her as a goddess, a symbol of female charm, my dream. And she looked at me as if I was a god. I felt if my plans worked out she could be mine. When my companion and I caught the bus back to Lancaster University I again felt almost complete. But if I wasn't I now harboured the very real hope that soon I would be.

The end of term arrived and I boarded the train home with a mixture of hope and doubts as regards for what lay in store for me. Would I get the Christmas present I so desired? At Honiton station my mother picked me up and drove me home to our redbricked vicarage. At home neither my parents nor my sister mentioned my plans. They probably all hoped the whole idea had passed from my mind. But in the January, after a peaceful and reasonably happy holiday, I suddenly announced I was going by train to London to have my nose done. I prevailed upon my reluctant father to lend me the money towards it and I made that reckless journey.

After a hectic trip through London I arrived at Dr. H.'s clinic. I was shown into the waiting room by a grey-haired nurse.

Dr. H. made his appearance. He was dressed in a white coat and surgical hat.

"You are tall and good looking" he said. "Why do you want to have something done to your nose?"

"I want to realise my full potential " I replied.

"What would you like done to it?"

"I am slightly self-conscious about the left profile. I don't want the bone fractured." I had said all I thought necessary.

He left and almost immediately the auburn-haired nurse who had taken my photograph entered the room. It was strictly down to business and certainly she was leaving me no time to change my mind. I felt relatively optimistic about things at that moment and certainly was not on the point of that.

"Have you got a cheque for £300?" she asked.

"Yes" I replied and handed her the cheque for that amount. It was not too difficult a thing to do and to me it might as well have been just a bit of paper I was handing her. Exchanging bits of paper for the perfect face was how I saw it.

The nurse asked me for another cheque for accommodation during my recuperation and I handed over another meaningless bit of paper, paper at least meaningless to me. The nurse having accomplished what she wanted, namely the acquisition of those two bits of paper which were important to her if not me, left. I sat down in a chair twiddling my thumbs waiting for the inevitable. A little later the inevitable came closer with the entrance of the grey-haired nurse.

"I have bought you a couple of sedatives" she said. "We always try and relax patients before an operation." I was handed the sedatives on a tray which I dutifully swallowed helped down by a pot of water. The nurse told me to wait and again disappeared.

Ten minutes later she reappeared. By this time I was beginning to feel a little drowsy. I was told to get up and gently led upstairs to the room where Dr. H. had first interviewed me. Going up I felt a little unsteady on my feet. Upstairs I was asked to strip to the waist. Then I was led to the alcove containing the operating table and asked to lie down on my back. I was not aware of any instruments and the atmosphere was made to seem as innocuous as possible. There was not even the atmosphere of an operating theatre. Dialogue between doctor and patient was encouraged. I had been told that for convenience sake I would be given a local anaesthetic rather than put under. I was aware of Dr. H. bending over me and a painful prick as the needle was stuck into the tip of the nose. After that I could only imagine what was going on.

A little later the auburn haired-nurse returned. By this time the nose was starting to swell.

"I did not think it needed doing" she said observing my nose. "But looking at it now it probably does."

The doctor and the nurse both started to chat though I was not sure how much of their conversation was purely spontaneous and how much was designed to reassure the patient. They talked of the horror, of Nazi Germany and the extermination camps as if they were in the business of caring, the antithesis of Nazi Germany. They also raised the question of my personal life which they both seemed interested in. In addition the nurse's later words did suggest I would be truly handsome afterwards and Dr. H. had already said that in accordance with general practice if I was not satisfied with the nose he would do it again, something I was to bear in mind.

Two hours later, though I couldn't be sure of the time, I became aware of a black thread out of the corner of my eye. Throughout I had displayed a deep curiosity as to what was happening to me even though I had been advised to keep my eyes shut. I now experienced a sharp pain and had to grit my teeth. My nose was being stitched up. It was then totally covered up and I put my shirt back on.

I was helped up, led to an armchair and told to rest. The pain had not bothered me much, my only anxiety was whether or not I had achieved my ambition, whether or not I had the perfect nose. It was entirely my self-image that mattered and I had no inclination to rest though I had to remain seated in my armchair for an entire hour while a vain search for a taxi to take me to the accommodation address was made. Eventually Dr. H. and I set out on foot. We had about a mile to cover and it was quite an experience for as we walked down the pavement I noticed people looking in amazement at me with my heavily bandaged nose.

We arrived at the accommodation address which was fairly plush inside and took the form of a three bedroomed flat. There were several women in nighties and dressing gowns strolling about, some with covered ears or noses and some with noses that had recently been uncovered. Although I was slightly shortsighted, the results of the uncovered noses did not seem too bad from the distance. I had no means of gauging how good Dr. H. was with mens' noses for there were no other male patients there. It is easy for a man to know what is beautiful in a woman, but it is not so easy for him to know what is handsome in a man.

Before I could effect a detailed inspection of my flat mates I was led into a room that was actually used as a lounge where there was a camp bed. I was told all the beds had been taken in the bedrooms, but being a man it was assumed I would not mind roughing it and indeed I had no objection to that.

For the next three days I had only one thing on my mind – noses. I had not imagined at first that there would be very much to having a rhinoplasty. One of the two nurses had said that in my case only a very simple correction was needed. But I still dreamed and still I prayed. I didn't know if I was more concerned as to whether I would look worse or whether I had received that spur to conquer the world, to conquer at least my own self-doubt and reach that pinnacle of experience, an ideal love. The three days passed very slowly.

At last the time came to have the coverings removed and the stitches taken out and I walked back to the clinic with Dr. H.. In the upstairs room I was asked to lie down on the operating table. The light was directed over my face making me blink. The stitches were then removed, a painful procedure though I was not worried by the thought of physical pain. It was only mental anguish that held any terrors for me. It was an anxious few minutes. The moment of truth came. I was told to get up.

That I did with as much dignity as possible making my way slowly but surely to the wall mirror. I had been told the nose would end in a point and to all intents and purposes that was how I wanted it to end. When I looked in the mirror I was greatly shocked.

My nose was bulbous and greatly swollen.

Downstairs the grey-haired nurse noted that I was not my normal cheerful self. Now was the moment of reckoning and a deep feeling of sadness had come over me. Clearly I had lost a certain of my radiance and things had gone slightly wrong. The nurse assured me that the swelling would go down and that it would turn out a lovely nose, but I was not sure that I fully believed her. "All the girls will be after you" she said. I could not honestly believe that what she said would be the case and all I really wanted was happiness. I did not necessarily want to be worshipped.

I picked up my few belongings and left the clinic a changed person. I followed the underground to Waterloo station and then caught the train back to Devon conscious all the time of being somehow different, conscious of the people looking at me. And they were looking at me for I was a spectacle with my deformed and enlarged nose. I was a monster. Going about looking as such did take inward courage. As such I would be ostracised, I would be an object of curiosity. But I was basically optimistic about life and though my hope of achieving my dream had been set back I believed time was the healer, the swelling of my nose would go down and that I would fit back into society. I had only ever considered what it would be like to be divine. I had never considered what it would be like to be the opposite, horribly ugly. The maimed and disfigured had before only been peripheral to my existence. I could now glimpse what it must truly be like to be one of these unfortunate people. But my humiliation seemed only temporary and I hoped I would soon emerge from my present grey world into broad daylight again.

At home I asked my sister what she thought of my new nose.

"Well , I couldn't see anything wrong with the first one" she replied.

I realised she was incapable of understanding me and my aspirations or the obstacle I saw to achieving my aspirations and that I was confronted with the problem of people misinterpreting me and my actions. This problem was not so bad at home for my sister had some idea of my former attractiveness particularly as a boy. But the misunderstanding of me by those who thought they understood me when they didn't would spread through my life like a cancer. The change now was such that anyone knew me closely would see it, a change for the worse. People who thought they knew me but in fact didn't would read into it not only my present failure but a failure in the past, a failure that had never really existed. Had my gamble been successful I would have been respected. Now I had been shamed.

I still had ten days to go till I returned to Lancaster University. In that time my face could settle down, I could approach what I had been, my self-confidence could mend, at least enough to get by. I prayed for improvement, all round improvement, improvement both physically and emotionally. All I could do was pray. And my face did settle down, not as much as I would have liked, but a bit.

On my return to Lancaster University I was terribly shy and nervous that people might notice a change in me. I wasn't the monster that had returned to Devon on the train immediately after the operation. But I was changed. No one said anything and on that score I was relieved. But other shocks awaited me. The worst was that none of the belles in the university appeared to notice me anymore. I had lost some of my magic, I no longer had any power or influence left to make my way with the beautiful, to determine what was good for me and what I felt was appropriate not only to my needs but my aspirations.

Shortly after my return to Lancaster University I decided to move from campus to digs in Morecambe. Perhaps I hoped that by returning to Morecambe I might be able to recapture that sense of freedom that I had experienced on my first visit there, that day of true happiness. I was too vulnerable on the campus, too exposed to people, people who now looked upon me and treated me differently, notably the beautiful whose affection and regard could be so drastically affected by a simple alteration to one's nose. In moving to Morecambe I was in effect running away, even if I was running away as much as anything from myself. In going there I hoped to rediscover happy associations. But it was just another disaster. I arrived there on another cold day, but it was not only cold, it was grey. I found digs in a Victorian terraced house, one room but not uncomfortable. The town itself came across as a lonely and bleak place and the sea was an angry dark colour on my arrival. My next humiliation came when I bumped into my love goddess on a bus. She it appeared also had digs in the town. And she did not even look at me let alone as if I was a god.

A day or two after my arrival in Morecambe I went to a student party in the town. I was anxious to make friends for although I could stand loneliness I did not relish it and in my predicament it was difficult not to be lonely. The party was held on the ground floor of another Victorian house. There was a vast preponderance of male students, mainly drunk, though there were a few females. In one darkened room the numbers were about equal and I went and sat down on the floor. A record player in the room was giving forth some sleepy erotic music and I got talking to a girl, an American. Then the lights came on and the girl I saw was only ordinary. Even she seemed to lose interest in me. I had a painful, even tragic glimpse of my own acquired insignificance.

Meanwhile exams or at least one exam loomed up for that January an Economics exam had been set for the first year group. I was admittedly depressed but that did not stop me applying myself for my exam. I was fortunate in that I had a marvellous set of school notes on Economics and I simply swatted up on these so when it came to the exam I had no difficulties. Apart from this I was unable to study properly. At school I had enjoyed working but now my studies, particularly Mathematics, became a burden. I needed help and yet it is at such times that people shun you. Sadness must be endured alone. I still continued to attend lectures, and in the English seminars I stared straightfaced at the lecturer completely ignoring the other students as they ignored me. I was shutting out the world and single-mindedly going about my own business, plodding on alone to what seemed the questionable goal of academic success. At the same time I still hoped that my nose would get better even more and indeed it did but so imperceptibly I hardly noticed. During one Maths lecture I suddenly broke down. I couldn't walk out of the lecture for I would be to conspicuous so I did all I could to hide my tears; I buried my face in my hands. When the end of the lecture came the tears still came and my eyes were visibly red and swollen. All I could do was to remain seated and try and hide my tears. The students all filed past me looking at me and my humiliation was complete. It was stupid even trying to carry on.

That same day I set in motion the procedures for leaving, for abandoning my chance of being successful and respected. But I was surrendering my chance for academic success with dignity. I might even be given another chance. And I was doing the only

50

thing I could do. So with more relief than hesitation I wrote off letters from my little room in Morecambe to all my lecturers and the university authorities informing them I was leaving. The next day the people concerned received the letters and sent back notes urging me to stay or at least to come back the following year. I saw my tutor that same day and said something about wanting to give up Mathematics and to take up Politics instead. That was not possible nor indeed was it really the issue so I returned to my digs, packed my bags, paid off my landlady who was indignant that I had only taken a room for two weeks, caught a bus to Lancaster then the next train to London.

CHAPTER 3
LONDON.

I arrived at Euston station with my bags and suitcase unsure of what to do or where to go. I had not planned my departure from Lancaster University very well. I was just blindly escaping. But at least I had escaped from an existence that was proving to be a problem. Now I had arrived in London, the place where Dick Whittingdon had gone, made his fortune and become Lord Mayor. I didn't expect to be Lord Mayor but I did believe in London I could find a refuge, even respectability. I thought like many who converge on this grand metropolis that I would find something better. The bright lights are an attraction to a soul in distress. They promise to populate a lonely heart. You don't expect to feel alone amidst nine million people.

However standing on the platform at Euston station I was very much alone even if I didn't realise it. It might have seemed a simple question of looking up the accommodation column for a flat and the job column for a well-paid career. I had three A.levels and a clean record so what was stopping me? But life is not so simple and London was a far tougher place than that. The unemployment figures were beginning to rise and accommodation was scarce and costly. I was battling against odds I didn't appreciate. I had suffered the rigours of boarding school but had always been cushioned by the thought that I was being equipped for the modern world, for comfort, prestige, wealth and respectability. The real world and what it implied had not yet sunk in.

So alone I stood on the platform of Euston station with my bags and suitcase and nothing, nothing except two addresses both of old school friends. One was Jerome and the other an Indian friend who had digs in Streatham Common. I decided to make my lonely way to Streatham Common to the abode of my Indian friend.

I arrived at the house in a street in the second stage of decline. Parked outside a few of the semi-detached houses and untended gardens were some old jalopies, the symbol of declining affluence but the street was not quite a slum and had potential. I walked up the pathway to the front door and pressed one of the buzzers. It was beginning to get dark and it was the hour that commuters returned from the centre of the grand metropolis to their suburban homes. I waited for a reply but no one came to the door. I was beginning to wonder if I had made a mistake, if my journey to this far-flung and seedy part of London had been in vain, when a girl who happened to be opening the door of the house next door asked me over the hedge who I was looking for. She was like an angel of mercy at that precise moment and I gave her the name.

"Oh he's probably at the pub" she said. "I'll take you there."

The girl was called Joyce and was both very pretty and kindly looking with auburn hair. She was the first warm heart I encountered and a warm heart with implications.

At a pub nearby we did meet up with my Indian friend who was at the bar drinking shorts. He was now at the London School of Economics doing no work. He was aged before his time in his view of life and exploited his youth and good looks with a liberated zeal. Indeed he had only to respond for he was one of the lucky few to whom women made advances and it was but for him to slight or embrace. Joyce had first approached him and attracted by her femininity and European charm he had responded.

He quickly finished his short and we three made our way back to his bedsit. He only had one room and the house inside was cold, damp and miserable. There were no curtains and the toilet was shared with two others, both West Indians. I wasn't sorry for my friend, only for the West Indians and myself; we were impoverished. And my Indian friend as I discovered, hardly ever slept in his dark hole. He nearly always slept in a foreign bed in more congenial surroundings. But I now at least had a roof over my head for which I was grateful and a base from which to plan my new life.

That same evening I wrote off to my parents informing them that I had left university and that I was in London. I knew it might be considered a cowardly action writing such fraught letters to my parents but I knew I could not bring myself to face them about such important matters. I did not expect them to understand. And what might seem right or reasonable at this stage did not fit in with my emotional state which I thought was always the most important consideration.

The next day I visited Joyce in her bedsit next door with my friend. She lived in a house a shade more commodious than the house in which he lived and her room was very comfortable in comparison to his. There was a kitchen unit with fairly up to date appliances, clean, white and well-lit, divided from the rest of the room by closing doors so as not to spoil the impression of a bedroom. The floor was carpeted with thick pelt, there was a fur rug on the double bed and a coloured television set. Before I left that evening she gave me an invitation to come round whenever I liked, an invitation that in my Indian friend's dark, cold, unfriendly room,I could hardly refuse.

Two days after my arrival my friend told me that he and Joyce had had a disagreement about sex and that he had decided not to see her for a week. He told me to inform her of his decision. I was not aware of the rights and wrongs of the matter but knew he could be slightly heavy handed and I rightly or wrongly tended to sympathise with Joyce. So I made my way over to her bedsit partly with the intention of telling her what he intended, but principally to seek the warmth and comfort of her room for I was fed up with the squalor in which I was living. Joyce had just returned from work. She was a secretary for the BBC. I mentioned what my friend had said but in a way that would not cause her unnecessary pain. It was then that she started to be very warm towards me, and her warmth gave me hope that my nose might not be so bad after all. I thought of my friend and I wondered what future there was between Joyce and him but I was not particularly worried about that. Certainly life did not give him cause for any deep worries.

Two days later I received a reply to my letter to my parents. My father had written an encouraging letter designed to get me to have a rethink about my decision to leave Lancaster University. He said that my Economics tutor had written to say that I had done extremely well in the Economics exam coming top of his three groups with an A and that Lancaster University did not like to lose good students. I was told I had two weeks to come back. But I was still very insecure and did not feel I could face all those students again or the unhappiness of my last few days there.

My friend did not return that night nor the following evening; no doubt he was making other conquests and living it up in the style to which he was accustomed. On both occasions, feeling uncomfortable and a little lonely, I visited Joyce. She asked me: "Are you a virgin?" "Are you trying to save yourself up for something?" I was not promiscuous and analysing my mind would have liked to wait till I met the person I planned to marry before losing my virginity. And as said through fear of failing I was anxious to put off this moment. On this occasion though there was no backing out. I was just too vulnerable and weak to resist. I was perched on the edge of Joyce's bed on the fur rug and Joyce had seated herself close to me. I saw her hand move to the buttons of my shirt and then to the buckle of my trousers. Not a word was exchanged. Before I knew it both she and I were naked, our clothes in an untidy pile at my feet on the floor. There was no going back. Whether I liked it or not I now had to complete the ritual. This was to be a test of my remaining worth in the eyes of female kind.

I viewed Joyce; she had stood up in front of me a little way from the bed; she had the body of a girl all white and delicate.

"Do you like me ?" she asked.

"Yes" I said and we stepped into bed.

At that moment I wondered what this fragile girlish creature could offer me. I now regarded myself as in need of support. How could she support me when her appearance suggested that she was the one who needed support? I was not even sure that she was my type of woman. But at least she recognised me as some sort of a man. I asked her if she was protected.

"I'm on the pill" she replied.

54

She seemed on the whole a sensible girl who did the sensible thing. With that thought I penetrated. I felt a sudden surge of excitement then it was all over.

"Don't worry" she said. "That happens to most first time."

At least she was sympathetic, but if only I had been the man I had been at fourteen. But though I had experienced nothing of the ecstasy I thought was normal I had taken that step into the world which I had feared through anticipating failure. Had I been rejected at this instance my self-confidence would have been shaken and the future would have seemed formidable. But that was not the case and the next bit of interesting news was that my friend had made the same mistake, repeatedly. With Joyce at least, he was a failure in bed.

At the end of the week my friend, true to his word, said to me that he was going to see Joyce and asked me to tell her this which I went and did. I had mixed feelings about him coming. The idea did not fill me with dread but curiosity as to what Joyce's reaction would be. Shortly after my arrival at her bedsit there was a knock at the door and my friend entered. He mumbled something about my leaving in his usual self-assured tone. He was confident that Joyce would have learned her lesson and that she would be only too eager for any sort of affection from him. I was not going to try and come between them and thereby make a fool of myself so I tentatively got up to go. But as I was doing so Joyce exclaimed to my friend:

"Why don't you go and Andrew stay?"

My friend stalked out of the room.

This was like a small victory for me and an opportune one. I began to feel that whatever I had suffered to my nose not all was lost. And my friend, who at least was always very pleasant to me, went off and met a beautiful Indian girl who was perhaps more appropriate for his needs than Joyce.

I had thought about getting a job and had been to the job centre looking at all the advertisements pinned up on the notice boards. I scanned the job columns in the Evening Standard. There was an advertisement for a management position offering American rates of pay. It sounded hopeful. I rang up the number given and went to an interview in Central London along with fifteen others. Most of us were provisionally granted a job and asked to turn up the following Monday. It was then that I tried to establish the true nature of the job but as usual, when asking if it involved door to door selling, I was fobbed off. Needless to say two days later we all found ourselves being driven out by the carload to Croyden where we each had to canvas two or three blocks. The job was selling investment policies for which I had be given the patter to practice on clients but however impressed they were with the patter, clinching the sale proved another matter. As the evening advanced the rain started to fall worsened by a sharp gale that lashed at my legs and totally soaked if not totally dispirited I found myself huddled beneath the concrete steps of the garage annexe of a block of flats. It got worse rather than better and after a week I acknowledged defeat wending my way to the employment centre instead to peruse again without success the job advertisements on the notice boards.

Luckily I still had Joyce to brighten what might otherwise have been a rather miserable existence . She could be truly fun to have around. But one day I did become aware of a niggling little fault, to be precise, an excessively sloping shoulder, obtruding between me and a genuine love or appreciation. Our Indian friend had remarked upon it as well and it was the one thing that prevented her from being truly beautiful. However with my continuing anxieties and with nowhere else to go her warmth and encouragement were appreciated.

Regrettably I still had no funding coming in so I was obliged to make my lowly way to the social security offices for my area. I believed in the welfare state and though I had not availed myself of its benefits before I had an idealised view of this ideal. After the usual wait I walked over to the cubicle and sat down opposite the clerk separated from me by a contraption of wire and glass. I proceeded to explain that I had an education grant but that it still had to be paid back to my parents local authority. The reply was that as I had money handy I was not entitled to benefit. I had been deliberately avoiding Joyce for the previous two days so as not to give the impression of cramping her and I was feeling fairly isolated and what with my lack of success in practically every department of life I was beginning to feel like the archetypal failure. The road past the social security offices was both fast and dangerous and in a moment of black despair I walked across it hardly looking to see if any cars were coming, almost not caring if I was run over. It was the first time I had knowingly risked death.

Luckily after a further two weeks of following up advertisements in the local newspapers I succeeded in finding a temporary let in Tooting Bec, a convenient distance from Streatham Common with a ready bus service and I was able to escape the squalor of my Indian friend's room. The house was red-bricked, one of several in a reasonably prosperous middleclass neighbourhood and my flat was newly painted and carpeted, luxury I thought. By spending the remainder of my grant on a portable black and white television and radio record player I had everything to be comfortable again.

Almost straightaway I was also fortunate to get a job with a finance company. I was a little dismayed that first day in the office when my immediate superior presented me with several ledgers of bad debtors going back over many years and then set me to work writing letters threatening court action. A day or two later the manageress, a large battle-axe of a creature, also made me go out with my immediate superior in his car to confront bad debtors face to face. I had a vision of an ugly doorstep confrontation with a gesticulating near lunatic. Instead we arrived at one of my superior's houses undergoing renovation for resale, his way of supplementing his meagre income as a debt collector, but whatever the unpleasant aspects of the job I was now at least able to eat and to pay the rent.

With a place of my own I was now also in a better position to repay the hospitality bestowed on me by Joyce and I invited her over for a meal to my flat regaling her with spaghetti bolognaise carefully prepared in the kitchen next door, something I repeated more than once. Our main topic of conversation was the interrelation of the sexes. We started with my Indian friend and it emerged that his reason for wanting to chastise Joyce was that she had teased him about his sexual performance. Obviously their breakup had been a two way thing. I also ascertained that Joyce hated emotional men and that she found cruel men appealing. Fortunately, despite my previous harrowing experiences, I avoided any show of emotion. I did even behave rather cruelly to Joyce making her cry more than once to ensure her respect. But all the time it was as if I was behaving against my true nature and beliefs. Certainly in my innocence I didn't appreciate that it might have been those very beliefs that were inhibiting me sexually. Though I was occasionally hard the pull was usually towards being kind and compassionate and thus away from the chance of this brand of success.

On the employment side not only did I not have the Fascist mentality necessary to be a successful debt collector but I got paid so little I was virtually living hand to mouth. In addition the manageress decided to offer to teach me the job, something I stupidly accepted. She showed me how one type of voucher worked and when I asked her to show me how another type of voucher worked she claimed she had just shown it to me and in her office suggested that I resume my studies. I resigned my post and left with two weeks pay.

After my resignation from the finance company I said to Joyce that I might go to France then I decided to go home for a weekend without inviting her; she was deeply offended.

"Why won't you take me home to your parents?" she demanded. "Are you ashamed of me? Am I not educated enough for you?"

"No" I replied.

"If you loved me you would have been only to happy to introduce me to your parents."

A long time previously, in my dim distant past, I had made a decision that the only person I would bring home to my parents would be the girl I was going to marry. I did not envisage marrying Joyce so I went home to my parents without her. Indeed it was almost as if I was engineering a break up with her. It was a relief to get away to the countryside where I could be with my parents, sister and two cats. It was only to be expected that in my absence Joyce should go out and find someone else. That fact was perfectly apparent to me when I returned.

The following week I brooded somewhat and even sent Joyce a letter. She had at least provided me with an element of security and for me it was as if my anchor had been cut and I had again been left to drift on the rough seas of life alone.

But now I had my excuse to leave London and I applied for a place to read French at St. David's University College, Lampeter. The university only had six hundred students but I thought it would be more homely than Lancaster University. The previous year my old English master's son had been president of the students union there and had recommended it. The day of my interview was both warm and sunny and the lecturer beaming down at me through thickframed spectacles accepted my French was rusty and I was accepted on the spot. I prayed that by the time the new university year started I would have it in me to study again. In order to polish up my French I then got a job as a courier with Canvas Holidays. The courier party was to leave the following Friday.

A couple of days before I left I downed two or three pints of cider in my flat with the intention of fortifying myself for conquest. I still had this need to prove myself and thought that a regular diet of different women might help me to forget myself and provide me with meaning. So when I was sufficiently drunk I caught a bus to Croyden and went to a disco called Jacks. In the semi-darkness I slumped down at a table opposite two sisters. As my eyes got used to the flashing red, blue and yellow I saw that one was very pretty the other ordinary. She was grossly inebriated but very lively. After about five minutes she grabbed hold of my arm and whisked me onto the crowded dance floor. This pleased me as I had hoped to meet an ordinary girl rather than a pretty one so as to be sure of success. We chatted amiably and then she invited herself back to my flat.

There on some cushions on the carpeted floor we lay entwined. She rose claiming that that evening she had spilt something on her jeans and that they were wet asking to take them off. I didn't object and she then proceeded to seduce me. Very soon after entry I felt ready for emission so I suggested we move onto the bed. By some careful control I even managed to extend the act to a full fifteen minutes but it had been fifteen minutes of rather boring hard work. It would have taken time to perfect my technique but at least I had not made a fool of myself. Though the incident did have the effect of taking my mind off things there had been no emotional connection and when I put the girl on a bus to Croyden the next morning she passed out my life almost as if she had never existed. It didn't help when a day or two later I felt an ache in my testicle and had to make my embarrassing way to the doctor's surgery. There was a slight swelling for which I was prescribed antibiotics and I was left with marginal right epidydimusal expansibility. I concluded that one night stands were a waste of time but those capable of fulfilling me were beyond my reach it seemed. I remained mixed up.

The day before I left London my parents came up by car from Devon to collect my things and we spent the evening in the West End. Over a meal I explained my grant position and my father agreed to pay it back. We then went to see Carte Blanche. The writer of the play obviously had a phallic fetish for the male players spent the whole evening parading round the stage sporting phalluses of ever increasing proportions to the excited exclamations of the female players. After the show my parents and I went for a drink in an expensively furbished pub. That evening I had dressed in my navy blue suit and stacked shoes. My suit padded me out and gave me a strong manly appearance and in the pub I noticed a very pretty blond staring at me. When my parents and I finished our drinks and left I noticed that the girl's eyes were pursuing me out of the pub. It had been an amusing evening and I realised that in my navy blue suit I still enjoyed English good looks. Obviously a muscular appearance was some compensation for a damaged nose.

The next day I left London, Joyce and the bright lights for France and a new life. In Paris where I was putting up tents I found myself thinking about Joyce. I continued to the Loire where I put up more tents, this time in pouring rain. Here again I felt miserable. My third and last port of call was Touques in Normandy and here I settled down fractionally. I occupied a luxury tent much along the lines of those used by other holiday makers with Canvas Holidays and I was also provided with a mobilette enabling me to tour the surrounding countryside of green fields dotted with half-timbered houses and apple blossom filled orchards. Here I got to meet people in particular a small sprightly French girl of about sixteen. I had been relaxing bare-chested in a deck chair soaking up the hot Normandy sun when I noticed her staring at me. The next two days she kept on appearing. She even walked round the campsite with me as I checked tents. A friend commented what a pretty girlfriend I had though I did not see her as beautiful; I liked women of average build and along with underlying doubts was a continuing memory of Joyce.

But though I was preoccupied with matters of love I still retained some of my childhood fascination for warfare and castles and I took some of the holiday makers with Canvas Holidays to see a castle in Touques built by William the Conqueror. It was largely in ruins but still had the flavour of a heroic past. I recalled that at Eye when I was just nine I had wanted a suit of armour for Christmas and had got a tennis racquet. I was annoyed. It was amazing how ideals could alter.

On my eventual return home I found a letter waiting for me from Joyce. It was chatty but uninformative and I did not reply. At home I felt unproductive and the lack of activity allowed me to brood even more. Of course I still had to fit back into village life but fortunately my nose went unnoticed. After a service one Sunday, an attractive girl who was visiting the area, took a deep interest in me. At the time I was dressed in my navy blue suit and stacked shoes. Her attention warmed my heart. Most of the time I did feel pretty uninspired and lacking in incentive and though I did read L'Immoraliste, a set book, I was not operating at peak. I determined that I would have to come out of myself, meet people and in accordance with my instincts pursue those who did have the qualities to fulfil me though as more mature I would have had no problem relating. In my suit I would, as in the past, stand out. It was with this thought that I approached going back to university though, despite months of self-doubt, I could have had no idea of the awful suffering I was about to let myself in for.

CHAPTER 4
DREAM FRAGMENTED.

I was driven to Lampeter by my father. It was late September 1977. On the way I recognised much about the countryside, town and college that I had noticed on my first visit although in subsequent months the seasons had wrought subtle but significant changed upon everything. The sun that had shone so brightly no longer shone and the sky that had been blue had changed to an ominous grey. The rolling hills around Lampeter were not the pleasant green that they had been on my first visit, but also an ominous grey, an extension almost of the grey sky. It was not a day to warm my heart, but I still hoped Lampeter would provide me with the answer and that here meaning would be restored to my life.

At the college I got the keys to my room from the porters lodge and with my father's help carried my bags and case to my room which was on the second floor of Lloyd Thomas Hall. It was all very comfortable but as I entered the room I found my surroundings close in on me.

After my father left I had a look around the college to see what there was in the way of life. The main buildings modelled on an Oxford college and in the shape of a quadrangle were very attractive but I found little life, particularly female.

Luckily I did succeed in distracting myself a little later when I met up with two old school friends also starting at Lampeter. One was John who had stayed on an extra year at school to resit his English A. level getting a grade A this time, reflecting the subjective marking of such papers. He had a room on the middle floor of a hall of residence across the campus stream. The second friend was Steve, a calm sympathetic chap who still involved himself with other peoples problems and had a room on the ground floor of the same hall of residence. I was nonetheless averse to imparting any confidence to either about my recent history.

That evening after tea in the refectory, a building adjoined to my own hall of residence, there was a union meeting in the union hall chaired by Ray, the college union president. As at tea I did glance around in the hope of seeing a pretty face. None were evident and for someone who had formulated a philosophy of life based on pretty faces their absence was disconcerting.

The next day lectures started. I found that my reading of certain set books the previous holidays was a help and in normal circumstances I would have found the lectures enjoyable. Now as usual I was preoccupied with my private worries, although when I came to read over the notes I had made during the course of the day I discovered that I had absorbed more than I thought. In addition to

French, I was doing Greek and Roman Civilisation and English and I did hope that I would be able to concentrate enough to get through my first year.

About three days after the start of term I went to a disco in the union hall. John advised me strongly not to go. He had seen Ray dancing with another male on campus at a previous disco. As he spoke there was evident disgust in his voice. Disregarding his advice I went along but my search ran a blank. I truly wondered whether I hadn't arrived at the end of nowhere though I didn't give up hope of a pretty face appearing. I resolved to concentrate on my studies.

Two weeks into the first term a new first year student called Nick turned up. He was an extrovert and through him I was drawn into the social scene. We first met at a French lecture when noticing me in the corner he made a bee line. I was termed striking and he had singled me out. Nick was of public school extraction like me, short, stocky, regular featured and manly. He exuded warmth and charm which earned him a big circle of friends though they remained peripheral during our acquaintance. We spoke about everything and my confidences he accepted unthinkingly. His room was on the ground floor of Lloyd Thomas Hall.

One Friday evening about two and a half weeks after the start of term Nick and I went to a cheese and wine party in the university put on by the French society. Nick was dressed in a suede jacket and trousers and I was resplendent in my navy blue suit and stacked shoes. He was as confident as ever and I felt myself that I was still attractive to pretty women in my suit. I had also decided that what I had lost in looks could be made up for in character and I determined to put this the test. Some thirty or forty people were present at the party and behind a trestle table on one side of the room a girl was ladling out mulled wine into glasses. Nick and I walked over and helped ourselves to a glass. We looked round for examples of female beauty, but there were none.

However a little later my eyes fell upon a girl in a longish black dress by the trestle table, a pretty girl. "Look over there" I said pointing in her direction. "Yes, I see her" he replied. "Do you think she is pretty?" "Yes." The girl was blonde-haired, about five feet two inches tall and of medium build. She had a soft complexion, pretty confident eyes, a fine nose, and sensuous lips. In every way she conformed to my sense of form. I said: "She's the first girl I've fancied in this whole place."

After the cheese and wine party we decided to go to the disco held in the union hall. The pretty girl had also made her way there. The disco was beginning to fill up and I searched for her amongst the host of faces. I asked Nick if he could see her and he pointed her out. She had just finished dancing with an elegant young man. I had determined to take my chance with her and ask for a dance. Nick urged me to do just that but before I went over I asked him how I looked. "Fine" he replied. Anyway I was still confident in my suit so I went over to the girl and said: "May I have a dance with you?" "Well you may do after the next two " she replied. "I'm booked up till then." Her voice was like the tinkle of a silver bell, and very refined. I walked off to await my turn. When it came a slow record was playing and I started to dance with her. She said: "You look handsome in your suit." "And you look very pretty in your black dress" I replied. "Thank you." Her flattery inspired confidence and I said: "I noticed you at the cheese and wine party." "And I you." We lapsed into silence, then she said: "It's hot in here. Shall we go out? Perhaps you can walk me back to my room?" But first we walked into town skirting the edge of the campus. The night was quiet and still and the streets were deserted. The girl was called Enid and she was in her fourth year. She like me was reading English and French and had just returned from a year in France teaching at a lycee. Despite a small age difference we discovered common ground everywhere. We stopped near a street lamp and she said:"You can kiss me now if you like." We embraced and kissed. She had a clean natural smell and her kiss filled me with desire, a desire born not of love but of appreciation, for love had yet to come, a desire over which I had a firm control. "My room is in the quadrangle on the first floor" she said a little later. She led me through the campus car park next to Lloyd Thomas Hall and through the still night up to the main building and up a rickety wooden staircase. She opened the door of her room. "Here we are." I sat on the edge of the bed, a springy bed draped with a crochet rug. "So you're a little first year" she said and she sat down beside me and put her arms around me. Before I knew what was happening we were kissing passionately side by side on the bed. I faintly believed it might be the start of something wonderful. She flattered me and displayed a charm and intensity that took me by surprise. I in turn flattered her and acted as if I too was in control of life. As both she and I were looking our best it could not but be true mutual appreciation. Yet just to be with her made me happy. When I left Enid said: "Come back tomorrow."

Walking back to my room I inevitably had some remaining doubts, but I had a glow in my heart.

When I woke up the following morning I had a few more doubts about Enid and myself. She had only known me in my suit and it was only in my suit that I now had true charm it seemed. I wondered if she would accept me otherwise. Was there such a thing as true love, a love that could accept imperfection in another? "Could I continue my act and win her heart even without my suit on?" But I had not gone this far merely to give up what I had gained. So after lectures that afternoon, having dressed in fawn

63

corduroys and a diamond jumper, I went up to her room. As I entered she said "hello" in her same beautiful voice from a corner of the room where she was standing in tight trousers and top.

"I thought I would come round."

"I expected you to come" she smiled.

Her sheer certainty sounded ominous and obviously she knew I must have been thinking about her. She no doubt had been thinking about me too but clearly she had a certain control over her men; she was like a queen in control of her subjects. I just hoped and trusted she was genuine and I resolved to keep my emotions in check lest they engulf and enslave me. We sat down together on the edge of her bed and looked at each other. I took in her pretty countenance. In the afternoon light of her room she had a rare loveliness. She had just those qualities that could awaken my emotions. I wanted to flatter her, tell her how lovely she looked. She was highly susceptible to flattery.

"You have such a fine mouth" I said. "You have beautiful eyes too." I continued to catalogue her good points which in the light of her room were sundry.

"And you must have lots of girlfriends" she said treating my flattery as the sign of an accomplished roue.

We started kissing. My own physical desire was not what it had been but her's grew all the time. We lay on the bed and she acted as if she wanted top devour me but because she was pretty it made it all somehow respectable. Suddenly I found her on top of me and I could feel her warmth. I still felt no earnestness but then she started to slide about on top of me dominating me in a gentle way. "It's fun doing this " she commented and I answered in the affirmative. I thought what we were doing was fun but I did not want to go any further and break the spell. At any moment my act could crumble. I could make a great mistake and it would be the end.

After two minutes we rolled onto our sides and continued to kiss oblivious of the time and the world.I had again discovered a strange joy in simply being with a person, a joy which proximity of flesh heightened. But still at the back of my mind was a fear of failure, that Enid would detect beneath the gloss of my enthusiasm someone still to grasp the basics. I had gone as far as I was prepared to go. After some two hours I said:

"God, the time flies. I must be off."

I rose and she reluctantly let me go. I had savoured my first moment of happiness for a long time. After leaving her I continued to treasure a pleasant memory of her that sustained me through the day and made it a pleasure being alive casting a glow over everything. The university had ceased to be the bleak place it had done on my arrival.

I visited Enid again on the Sunday and Monday. On each occasion I had to tear myself away both because she didn't want to let me go and because I didn't want to leave. On both days she spoke about her concept of heaven which was rooted in the physical. She expatiated on the beauty of orgasm particularly when crowned with love and she encouraged me to unclothe her and find out about her body; soon I had familiarised myself with every part of it. To some extent I was pandering to her idea of heaven and would slowly rouse her to a pitch till she would beg me to "screw" her but drawing away leaving her frustrated. She went on to paint a true picture of paradise with her words and illuminated my mind on what could be if only I would respond and take what was mine. I did not remove a single garment and never considered doing so let alone going the whole way.

On the Tuesday I went up to her room after lectures and she welcomed me in her usual lively manner. We lay down on her bed and started to kiss and laugh; I felt my resistance slowly weakening. She was becoming more of a pretty face to me now. My emotions were coming into play. She it seemed knew how long this process took in men, presumably through past experience. She was just waiting for the right moment to assert herself. Then she asked:

"What does your father do?"

"He's in the church."

"A vicar, oh my God."

The matter was clearly a big joke to her. She was defying me and changing her tack. Her questions pointed at an attempt to dismantle the foundations of my beliefs. Christianity offered an undeniable moral logic and I couldn't understand her amusement.

"Where do you come from?"

"Originally from South Africa."

"Oh I met some South Africans. I hated them."

Her answer made me feel a little insecure. With this and further questions she was trying to make clear her selectivity over friends and lovers thus raising my estimation of her. She was making sure that I thought her the most precious being in the world; she made it seem as if there was no replacement for someone like her. Her questions continued. After all that she asked:

"Will you marry me?" She gazed into my eyes with a loving and angelic look as if she was asking for the world, as if I owned the world. It might have seemed the supreme moment of my life. I replied prompted more by insecurity than joy:

"I would marry you before any other girl in the world." Though I meant what I had to say I did not believe that she had meant what she had just said. But I suddenly realised that I was truly in love though the realisation only made me sad for I sensed the end, the end when the beginning was promised. My sense told me that happiness was too precious a thing for some to keep hold of. It was a fragile luxury. However, despite my doubts, I would have followed her to the ends of the earth.

I rose and left keeping my doubts to myself and she consumed my thoughts for the rest of the day. Before I might have been able to face her, but that sharp edge that she had revealed to me that day about the other side of her character cut into me for my nose still made me insecure. Did she really want to marry me?

The next morning I woke with continuing doubts but in a restrained way I did enthuse about Enid to John whom I visited that morning.

"I've met the most beautiful girl" I said. "So good, clean and nice." Even then I did not believe she was the genuine article. But I had give all the crucial details and did not want to discuss her anymore. What I was experiencing was too personal to share with my friends. I could only give hints of my inner world of experience. I could not permit my friends to step right into it. My desire for privacy in my personal life had always been with me and I had no intention of making my personal life public now.

On the Wednesday afternoon I could not face being away from Enid anymore.I had been thinking a lot about her and in order to calm a troubled heart I went up to her room for the fourth time. She had just arranged to go for a jog with some friends, but I did have a chance to glimpse her from close up again in her room. She was dressed in a cream track suit and at that moment in the shades of the afternoon I thought her the most beautiful thing I had ever seen. The sight made me feel insecure for I wondered how I could cope with such good looks and when I made to leave I was obviously miserable. She asked me to come and visit her that evening as if to reassure me and she followed me out of her room down the stairs into the quadrangle on her way to meet her running companions. There she came up to me and again reassured me.

At the steps to the main building she broke ahead but kept turning round and smiling at me. But as I made my way back to Lloyd Thomas Hall I still felt sad. Worst there was a hint of jealousy. This feeling increased when I saw her arrive at the spot where her running companions were and when she started to laugh and joke with them. It was the first time in my life I had been prey to such a thing. It retained a hold of me all the way to my room only going after she and her friends had disappeared.

That evening I went to the union bar with John and a couple of other friends and ordered a pint of cider. This I drank slowly and deliberately and after I had completed it I went and bought another pint which I also drank slowly and deliberately. After the completion of the second pint I felt I had enough confidence to go and see Enid so I got up from my seat and climbed the stairs to her room. I knocked on the door and she called me in. It was ten o'clock and she had been waiting for me.

I went and sat down in a chair by her desk and she came and sat on my lap. I felt her sumptuous body through my trousers and woolly jumper.

"You're wearing a jumper your mother knitted" she said in a beautiful maternalistic voice.

"Yes" I replied. She was very gentle and caressing and inspired by that I said: "You have no idea of how jealous I felt this afternoon." She smiled. "Do you hate emotion?" I asked.

"I think it sweet" she replied gently and coaxingly.

I let a tear run down my cheek. "We will be together till the end of the year won't we?"

"Of course" she replied.

After her marriage proposal I did not think that what I had asked for was unreasonable. Nine months of her life was all that I asked then if she wanted she could go and do whatever she pleased. She slid off my lap, made her way to the bed and pulled the mattress off the bedstead onto the floor. Having positioned the mattress on the floor she proceeded to undress.

"Well, come on then."

I had no choice in the matter so I in turn undressed. What I did not realise was that despite the previous exchange of words this was to be my great test. She lay back on the mattress her legs wide open. I lowered myself between them. What I feared might happen was happening. As I entered I felt myself hit against something rubbery. I assumed it was a diaphragm. Then I felt myself triggered on. I had experienced no build up and negligible desire. To avoid making a fool of myself I withdrew.

"Why have you taken it out?" she enquired.

"I'm about to come" I said sheepishly.

"Well come then." I did so. It was completely unsatisfactory.

Afterwards she said:"I don't feel the same about you anymore."

"I'll do better next time" I replied though I never wanted a repeat of this failure. And I knew it was the end as surely as death was the end. She had deceived me into thinking a stronger bond united us. But I was too miserable to be angry.

"Don't worry" she said. "Not all women are like me." Her words did not help. I was not interested in what any woman was like, only in what women like her were like. She turned away with a disappointed look on her face, as if I had let her down, as if she had experienced better. Her love for me had disappeared and a previous love, a consummated passion had been remembered. Her look only served to exaggerate my sense of failure.

She suggested we be friends. I felt friendship too great a compromise and I dressed to go. But as I was making to leave she started to reach out as if reluctant to let me go. I turned a blind eye to that and returned disconsolately to my room in Lloyd Thomas Hall.

CHAPTER 5
AN UNPLEASANT DREAM.

An hour later, dressed now in pyjamas and dressing gown, I returned to her room in search of reassurance. She was lying naked on the mattress and got up and embraced me. She pulled me down on the mattress and though I dreaded a repeat of the previous failure it inevitably came to entry. It was over almost immediately with her bouncing about on top of me in what I thought was a simulated orgasm. I was not reassured. She didn't want me seen there in my dressing gown and pyjamas the following morning and suggested I leave. Her voice sounded very final. I returned to my room and bed my dream in ruins.

That night I had difficulty getting to sleep so just lay in bed thinking. My thoughts rested principally with Enid and what had happened. I was doomed to languish. Hope had faded. I had looked upon her reaction to me as a mark of my own worth. Now she had pronounced her verdict. Unfortunately she had only done that after I had fallen in love with her rather than before. But I was more than ensnared by her now. I was ensnared by my own shortcomings. My chief ambition now was to overcome my shortcomings and so find my true mate and thus heaven.

At four in the morning I got out of bed, put on my dressing gown and sat down at my desk. I took out a writing pad from the top drawer and settled down to write a letter. I had been driven by my doubts to what seemed an act of desperation; I was writing to the Forum clinic, a sex clinic. It was something I wouldn't have dreamt of not long previously. The address I had found in the magazine of the same name. I hadn't bothered to write but now I filled eight pages. The letter was my first attempt to escape the snare.

The following morning I not only posted the letter but I broke my silence and told John, if not everything at least most things. Before Enid had boasted to her friends about me. I had maintained a faithful confidentiality about her. But as she had broken my trust I in turn broke her trust in me. I could not bring myself to tell John quite everything because I was naturally demure and I did not even mention the fact that she had asked me to marry her. But I was ceasing to care about personal dignity and words came more easily. Unfortunately to John my revelations pointed to only one thing- failure in life.

Later that morning, between lectures, I also visited Nick in his room and told him about the end of my affair with Enid mentioning my failure in the bedroom. This was the start of Nick's misunderstandings about me though he thought me reasonably good looking. Unfortunately he also had to listen to John's extreme views about me, they were in the same French group, and inevitably Nick's opinions were coloured.

In the afternoon, after lectures, still drawn by the fascination of Enid's room and a little encouraged by her expressed wish to be friends, I made my way up to her room to say hello. As I entered she looked at me as if she expected me, as if she had calculated my return.

"Why don't you write me poetry?" she said mockingly. "Plenty of people do."

All she wanted from me now was worship. She was like a Queen bee with all her drones buzzing around her. I wanted to own her, not just to be one of her drones, going on about how beautiful she was. Was that all I was good for? She went on as if poets and romantics were put on this earth merely to praise the great, successful and famous, adding that I had a romantic temperament. I had once wanted to be a poet. I momentarily thought of the fame of Lord Byron. My poetry was of this vein: "Hilaire Belloc has a big cock." I myself had only a millionth of a chance of being famous. I was destined to be a failed poet and my lot was praising the unattainable. After a few minutes of Enid's mockery I could take no more and asked:

"What do you like about me?"

"I like everything about you" she replied with a characteristic ambivalence.

She produced some photographs of her English boyfriend, her American boyfriend and her French boyfriend, all in bathing trunks. They were square and regular featured. She pointed out the occasional ripple of muscle. She praised their beauty and their sexual accomplishments to the heavens. She spoke as if they were perfect beasts put on this earth for her satisfaction.

"Why do you tell me these things?" I asked and she smiled. I wanted to ask her why she had bothered with me in the first place if she was only interested in types with physiques like Charles Atlas.

She said her French boyfriend used to get so excited when they made love that he would do it three times in a row and she lay back on her bed invitingly and seductively and smiled. I sat down next to her and tentatively ran one hand down her sternum as far as her stomach."If my French boyfriend knew what you were doing to me he would smash all hell out of you" she said and she went on as if her French boyfriend was not only capable of a fiery jealousy but that I was so weak and insignificant I wouldn't stand a chance.

"I hate your French boyfriend" I said. I felt no resentment, just very miserable, my misery spurred on by a sense of inadequacy at Enid's attempts to make me jealous in the face of what now seemed the unattainable.

"I'll try and find another man or woman" she said as if a pretty woman could do more for her than I.

"I should have been born a woman" I said sitting bolt upright on the bed.

"Yes, you should have" she replied making me feel that bit more inadequate. She went on to mock me about my notions of love smiling and enjoying every moment of it.

"How could she attack me like this?" I wondered. "Was it the right of women to kick a man when he was down?" I didn't like being punished for nothing. When I thought about it all I still really wanted were a few encouraging words. Her words had proved just one thing, poison. I resolved to have nothing more to do with her. As I made to go she said as if to perplex me more:

"Come back tomorrow."

The next day I woke up with thoughts of Enid and her words. When I went into breakfast I found I had lost my appetite and had difficulty swallowing my food. It was a clear case of unrequited love, a sickness that most people suffered from at least once in their lives, but a sickness which in my case the circumstances were totally unconducive to overcoming. My only hope was that as in the past, Enid, like the others in my life, would fade over time into insignificance. Such was my insecurity I was now even afraid to go up to her room.

During this time I attended lectures as usual, and in French literature I now began to discover a parallel between Enid's ideas on life and those of the writers I was studying. The French group was coming the end of L'Immoraliste by Andre Gide. I also had a glance at Les Mouches, a play by Sartre, which was my introduction to Existentialism. Solzhenitsyn defined Existentialism thus: As there is no God anything is permissible. I wondered if Enid's reading had reinforced her own atheistic views of the world. It was the fear that my whole Christian upbringing had been misleading that worried me the most.

By Saturday the temptation to see Enid became well nigh impossible to resist. It was not that my feelings were especially intense, just that I could not see an end to them. Again my primary desire and hope was to elicit a few words of encouragement. So far all she had said was: "You have such tremendous potential." But she had also run me down so instead of holding myself back I made my way to her room. I found her seated in the chair next to her desk. I was not sure how to approach her or quite what to say. Should I put on a hard front or should I get on my knees and beg for mercy. I knelt down in front of her and clasped her knees with both hands.

"Are you a masochist or something?"

I looked up at her. About her mouth hovered a cruel smile which would have rendered most girls ugly, a smile of contempt, but a smile that somehow made her even more desirable. I was curious as to why she took such delight in humiliating me, why she didn't just give me the few words of hope I required. I nearly asked her if she was a sadist. In the end I just asked her to kill me. She simply smiled her same cruel but now triumphant smile and asked me to get another girlfriend.

I left her room and headed for the disco in the Arts building. On the way I collected Nick. It was nine o'clock, early for a disco, and about six people were on the dance floor. The music was blaring and the flashing of coloured lights hid many a blemish on the faces present. I tried not to think of Enid's occasional beauty and thought of someone less striking as if looks had nothing to do with it. A mediocre girl with a fractionally receding jaw, pretty eyes, a slightly jutting nose and a curvaceous body outlined beneath blue jeans and a tea shirt came up to me.

"Will you rescue me?" she pleaded. I took in her appearance and observed, almost as if I couldn't help myself, that she was not as good looking as Enid. I said to myself: "No, it's not looks that matter, its purity of character. I must feast my eyes on the beauty of this girl's soul." I looked at the person from whom the girl wanted to be rescued. He had a resilient character I was to discover but a hooked nose got in the way of him being good looking. I decided to rescue the girl from the unprepossessing male though I was so upset by my encounters with Enid and so determined to vent my frustrations on anyone who came close to me that the girl would have done better to have gone off with him rather than me. We went onto the dance floor, did a few steps and embraced. After a second dance she invited me back to her room and we left the disco and made our way over the bridge across the stream to her hall of residence. She was called Linda.

In her room we lay down on the bed and started to kiss. Spurred on by the example of Enid who believed in instant action, I let my hand wander over her body. She pushed it off but I didn't despair letting it follow the same course it had done before.

"Are you a virgin?" I asked.

"Yes" she replied.

I established that she intended to remain that way till she was married. I thought her notion of chastity antiquated. It seemed so because Enid thought it as such. I allowed my hand to stray across her breasts feeling the nipples beneath her tea shirt. This time she did not remove it but she did say:

"I don't think you should."

"Okay, I'll go" I replied .

"No, please don't go" she pleaded.

This was the first sign of her giving in. Just a little more psychological pressure... But I had had enough and said:

"Sorry, it's getting late and I must go."

She said: "There's no need for you to go."

My true compassion manifested itself. Linda had no idea of my problems and the driving force behind my insensitive treatment of her. I agreed to remain. We talked endlessly and though she had a few things to recommend her she had only received one declaration of love and my interest remained minimal. Finally, at about three o'clock, I got away.

The next morning at her request I met her at breakfast. I discovered she was the leading figure amongst a gang of first year girls nicknamed the Muppets. When I appeared I found Linda in pride of place amongst the Muppets and I joined the happy band. Linda was perhaps the best looking of them and seemed proud of me.

After breakfast she invited me over to her room and when I came to leave she was again reluctant to let me go. I thought I saw in her that day the dawning of love and I found it a simple business to keep her not only interested but fascinated. Despite the fact that she, like Enid, had several admirers, she did not afford me the emotional relief I required. Nor did she distract me from my preoccupation with Enid. Lookswise there seemed a great difference and looks were the crux of the matter to me. Though I visited Linda a few more times that week Enid still occupied my mind. So the next Friday evening I returned to her room in the hope of obtaining some words of encouragement. Plucking up the courage to go and see her was very difficult. So far I had only succeeded once when I told her that I had, as she had suggested, discovered a little virgin and I was rather shocked by her attitude now for the first thing she said when I walked into the room was:

"Is your little virgin in love with you yet?"

Seeing that amatory conquests were just a game to her I walked out of the room disgusted.

A couple of weeks later I put on my navy blue suit and platform shoes and went to chapel sitting down in the green pews. chapel was not a mystical experience for me anymore. I just went as an excuse to put on my suit for I planned to see Enid after the service and I wanted to impress her and so at least get a warm word out of her for a world without love could be a cold unwelcoming place. I thought in a non-serious way that I might even ask her to help me sexually since it mattered to her so much. So all through the service my thoughts were not on God, as if he had ceased to be a reality to me, but of Enid and sex.

After the service she welcomed me into her room with open arms; obviously the suit made all the difference. I asked her if I could borrow her toothbrush and she acquiesced. Sharing someone's toothbrush was the most intimate thing I could think of because I was in fact sharing the bacteria in my mouth with her. After I had finished brushing my teeth I sat down on the bed next to her and we started to kiss. Soon she was hungrily seeking my body through my clothes. We did not attempt a repeat of what had happened before but she did "wank" me off, I was in control and performed expertly. Then I asked her if she could help me. To my surprise she agreed. After securing her agreement I got off her bed to leave and she rose and patted and smoothed my jacket.

As I walked out I realised that I had been in Enid's room for at least three hours though it had felt like five minutes. I also realised that we had been glorying in externals and certainly neither of us genuinely cared for the other. I also strongly doubted that she would go all the way and help me. But the fact that she had offered was a great boost to my self-esteem.

Lectures the next two days proved enjoyable in consequence and on each day after lectures I paid Enid a thirty second visit to find out if she was still enthusiastic. Just to feel that she regarded me as worth something made all the difference. I really just wanted an excuse for a tenuous link with her. I didn't necessarily have to own her. I just had to feel valued.

The next Wednesday morning as I stood in the breakfast queue with Digby, an army officer friend of John's, things took a turn for the worse. I had noticed Enid standing ahead of me in the queue and in sight of Digby, impelled by a sudden thought, I moved up behind her and threw my arms around her in what was intended as a gesture of friendship. She squirmed causing my arms to slip up to her breasts.

I released my hold, but she refused to acknowledge me. She had humiliated me in front of Digby. I saw that she had nothing left to offer me.

That same evening Enid noticed Linda and I sitting next to one another in the refectory lounge and she went red and stormed off. I had done precisely what she had told me to do in finding Linda. The next morning I received a letter scrawled in pencil from Enid. It was not written on letter writing paper but on foolscap and although she said I had potential to be all those things I "so desperately wanted to be" as if to be a Don Juan was my ambition, she also said I was "many light years away " from what she looked for in a man. I read it as the final rebuffal and the end of our relationship.

I began to feel tired of Linda. She might have been able to distract me before I met Enid but having been convinced that only through a person like Enid could I find true happiness and as she had described so vividly what she could do for a man, by associating with Linda I became ever more conscious of her theoretical shortfalls. I thought the best thing would be to stop visiting her or communicating with her but despite Enid's example of deliberate cruelty I was anxious to avoid causing her pain.

A little later Linda came up to my room. When I let her in she was in tears and obviously in a state of desperation: "Why haven't you been to visit me?" she asked. I was lost for an answer and receiving no reply she began to cry even more. I was touched. I had treated her badly up till now and such treatment had achieved the desired effect. But I intended to let her off more gently than I had planned. I would let the world think I was the reject, not her. I was not concerned with making endless conquests, purely with obeying my instincts in search of the ideal woman and as I was near to despair at this moment of achieving my ambition I didn't really care if people thought I was the reject. I was even content to run myself down in order to make Linda happy. So I said:

"If anyone asks you what happened just say you decided to end it all."

Neither John or Nick were ever able to grasp what truly happened between Linda and myself and they both thought I was the reject, not her.

As Enid had through her letter, severed all ties, she had again left me feeling miserable and empty. Study I regarded as sheer drudgery and in the Greek and Roman Civilisation lectures, the history of Ancient Greece passed before me as a meaningless blur as I sat at the back of the lecture theatre. My attending was fruitless.

A week or two later I got tipsy and paid Enid another thirty second visit. I made the visit merely to remind her of my existence though I certainly did not want to do anything more than remind her of it lest I disgust her as well. She was easily disgusted. When I arrived she told me to go to the disco being held that evening adding that there must be some young woman "dying" for me.

I thought now was the appropriate moment to forget about her and find someone whom I regarded as pretty. In the disco I looked around for a pretty face. My eyes fell upon a small attractive creature on the dance floor in a rugby shirt and jeans. She was much smaller than Enid, a small fairy princess. Enid said that she liked big brawny males. This girl being that much smaller would not require such brawn. She appeared to be dancing with a bearded male though she was standing several feet away from him looking about her all the time; obviously she was not taking him too seriously and I went up and asked her her name. It was Lorna. I asked her for a dance. She acquiesced. I established she was in her fourth year so evidently she was in Enid's year, and was probably reading French like Enid. I commented on her looks and she smiled. I jokingly asked her to marry me and she again smiled and went on enthusiastically dancing with me through the next two dances.

After the music of the third record had come to an end a very rough and ready third year student came up to me and said:

"Excuse me, but the lady already has an escort" and he pointed at the bearded male. I turned to him and said in a calm voice:

"Why don't you go to hell."

He persisted and in order to prevent a scene I decided to go outside with him. On the steps leading to the union hall the male gave his name. He then asked in a menacing voice:

"What are you playing at?"

"Nothing."

"Well unless you want your nose broken just carry on the way that you are."

"Break my nose then " I retorted for I was not the least worried by my nose, the cause of so much misery, being broken. Naturally surprised the male changed his tack and the evening ended up with a cup of coffee in his room.

Sadly that was not the end as I discovered when I went along to the next disco. It was again held in the union hall and as usual I was on the look out for a pretty face. Then I noticed a reasonably pretty woman in glasses sitting near the disc jockey operating the record deck and I went up to her and exclaimed:

"Christ, you would look ravishing if you didn't wear glasses."

At that instant, to my complete surprise, a dark figure rose from beside her. It was the same person I had met at the previous disco.

"It's not you again."

I didn't know what to say or do at that moment to mollify him. I just couldn't escape trouble. Then an angelic voice reached me from a secluded corner of the hall. It said:

"Come and sit next to me. I'll protect you."

The voice belonged to the lovely Lorna. She was like an angel of mercy. I had completely forgotten about her up to that moment. Now I gratefully accepted the offer. I knew she could not have objected to my extroverted behaviour before still to be talking to me now.

After about two minutes the bearded male appeared. She turned to me and said: "Let's go and have some coffee with friends" and she led me out of the disco to some lodgings in town. The bearded male I noticed was trailing behind.

I was led up to a room where three people were seated talking affably in armchairs. But I was not interested in Lorna's friends. I was under too much tension to start talking affably to people I hardly knew. I got up from the floor where I had been seated next to Lorna and descended the stairs. At the bottom I

76

noticed the door to the kitchen. The light was on and I entered. On the vinyl topped sideboard was an open packet of cream crackers and without thinking what I was doing but feeling the need to do something to relieve the tension like someone who bites their nails, I helped myself to two cream crackers and a tiny sliver of cheese from the fridge. I went upstairs again to the room where Lorna and her friends were seated. Not dreaming that I had anything to hide I offered one of the cream crackers to her and she accepted it happily. I started to nibble at the other. The whole thing remained a virtually unconscious reaction.

When Lorna and I left the sky outside was dark and the night still. The bearded male tagged on a few yards behind. I turned to Lorna and said:

"Will you kiss me?"

She just giggled and I did not press her. When I said goodbye to her she asked me where my room was and gave me precise instructions on how to get there. I left with a feeling of having witnessed someone very agreeable, but did not think of Lorna when I woke up the following morning.

Two or three days later I was confronted by the Heavy Brigade as I walked out of the refectory. The Heavy Brigade was an illicit organisation in the university created to ensure law and order. Its Colonel in Chief was the same chap I had met at the disco and was run under the auspices of Ray. The former called me over grabbing me by my scarf in a stranglehold forcing me to my knees in front of Nick and the other students milling around the refectory lounge. He then accused me of stealing food from people's kitchens. He must have been told that by Lorna. I was a little taken aback and assumed he must have been misled. He said I should see Ray.

A visit to Ray in his office in the union building caused me an even worse shock. Enid had made out I had "forced" my way into her bed, a total lie and she had wanted the Heavy Brigade to lynch me, all I assumed because I had paid some attention to the lovely Lorna and was jealous. Both Enid and Lorna, the latter spurred on by Enid's lies, had hatched a plan to blacken my name and destroy my reputation in the university. Enid for good measure had further tried to make out I had been pestering other female students. As I had only spoken to four girls I was a little confused particularly as they had not exactly been unwelcoming. But at least the Heavy Brigade had enough sense not to take the girls too seriously. Ray said of Enid: "She's snowed under with work" and advised me to steer clear.

A visit to Lorna's room, which was just below Enid's, helped to establish exactly what had been said. Nick was present on that occasion and Lorna was quick to realise she had been misled by Enid. Enid was summoned but with a brazen ferocity tried to justify her actions and was clearly annoyed or jealous that I had met up with Lorna which she obviously thought was a deliberate snub to her. It had been purely chance. Although Lorna did go on to scotch the rumours I was so sickened by Enid's approach not having then quite grasped the reason that I left returning to my room in Lloyd Thomas Hall throwing myself despairingly on the bed.

A little later Enid appeared along with Nick sitting down on the chair by my bed and taking hold of my hand. It soon became apparent that she was not there to make an apology. She simply brazened it out and further outlined my inadequacies going on to compare the strong athletic body of her French boyfriend with my own less formidable body. She made it seem as if it was a joke my going after Lorna because she was beautiful. In desperation I asked her to rate me out of ten so I knew where I stood with women. She gave me a rating of seven and a half out of ten without my suit on. I needed to be eight and a half or nine out of ten at least for what I wanted and I thought back to my nose mentioning having an operation. Enid thought the idea a joke. As soon as I raised the matter of her lies she rose and left with Nick following her out of the room. I gathered they went to the union bar then Enid invited Nick up to her room on the pretext of wanting to discuss me and then giving him an open invitation to visit her whenever he liked.

A few days later I wrote Enid a letter in response to her behaviour and her letter to me. As I didn't care about personal dignity anymore I did not hesitate to run myself down to emphasise what a mistake our relationship had been. It was a sort of self-destructive assault on her sensibilities. I said I would never be able to satisfy her large sexual appetite and that I lacked the brutishness and body she found essential in a man. I ended by saying that despite the fact she was a liar and a hypocrite I still wanted to be her friend.

No sooner had I placed the letter in her pigeon hole than I knew it was a mistake, that it revealed my own true despair . It had be the final throe in the agony of my ever growing awareness of my own inadequacy. I felt that after all that had happened I could never approach someone like her again. My life had generated into an unpleasant dream.

From then on I went progressively downhill; my behaviour in turn became affected though I could have perhaps got away with it had I not appeared so weak and vulnerable. One day I went into the union bar for a pint with Nick, sitting down opposite a handsome tall blonde-haired friend of Nick's called David who in turn was sitting next to a girl called Julie. At that moment Julie, who was of medium height and slightly tubby, opened her bag to extract something and I stupidly had a peep inside. She appeared annoyed at this and sick of people overreacting to me I started to empty it out for her. David remained unperturbed by events and did not look upon what I was doing with a critical eye. He was always calm and hardly ever critical of people. I soon stopped being silly hardly aware I had done anything terribly wrong. My first meeting with Julie resulted in her blackening my name to a few though I was so miserable I hardly noticed.

However I became very cynical about life and spoke at length to John about my cynicism even though he could conceivably have believed I was experiencing not cynicism but resentment. I felt no actual feelings of hostility and that would have been the honest observation.

It was at this time that I also described myself to John as "bewitched" and "under a spell", terms often applied to lovers and which I never literally believed but which would be thrown back in my face in the most devastating way at a later date.

I also spoke about my nose and I continued to wonder what could be done to it to give it that extra class that would increase my rating out of ten. I asked not only John but other people to rate me out of ten, and in turn my friends and I began to rate other students in the university out of ten on physical appearance.

All my preoccupations were a sign of my increasing personal insecurity. Although being a marathon performer had been an issue for a while now that I had met someone who put physical love above anything else, it came to matter more and more. This had all generated a phobia for rejection. Lorna would ask me to dance at the occasional social function but because my confidence had been so dented I always refused. She instead turned her attentions to Nick.

At last I received a letter from the Forum clinic in London asking me to attend and I hitched up to London arriving at the clinic at seven o'clock on a Friday evening. After half an hour I was shown into a room where two male therapists were seated and without being asked I sat down. I expressed my concerns to them but clearly they were not in the business of dealing out sympathy. It was their view I would have to learn to stand upon my own two feet and that was the only way I stood any chance of getting anywhere. I was asked if I was Jewish because of my nose and black hair and replied:"No." The therapists then got down to the real business asking me many intimate questions which were difficult to answer truthfully but which seemed to make sense. Having given the matter of sex a great deal of thought I began to feel more hopeful. One of the therapists asked me to draw my penis in its erect state on a piece of paper. I settled down to the unenviable task but such was my waning self-confidence I drew it about a quarter of its normal size.

"Is it that small?" exclaimed one of the therapists.

The next question was whether I was homosexual. I had thought about the matter a lot but gave what I believed was a truthful answer: "No." At the beginning of term at Lampeter University the Gay society had had a stand at the society gala where the students were invited to join the various societies and it hadn't entered my head to join. But it did seem to me at that moment that I must have descended a long way to be discussing the most intimate details of my private life especially as what we were discussing was in one way a joke.

The interview came to an end and I was grateful to hand over the £7, the cost of the session and to leave. I had four more sessions to go should I manage the trip up to London four more times, but the first was the worst and the worst was over. But I did have one or two nagging doubts for I expected to have to find a surrogate partner. The only advice I received was to alter or vary my grip during masturbation. It seemed as if I had to change purely through suggestion.

That night I slept in a hostel in Earl's Court and before lights out I wrote Enid a letter. It was well couched in contrast to my previous letter and said that I had seen a counsellor and that it was as if a dark angry cloud had lifted from my head. But I did add that after my experience with her I would have to fundamentally rethink my whole sexual outlook. I implied that sexual relations were a punitive experience, that she was a sexual vampire and that she had taught me the biggest lesson of my life. I worded my letter as an apology though it was really a vehement criticism of her conduct. I posted it the following day. I was however not remotely angry, just very miserable.

Even if I had hopes, a few days afterwards I began to feel that I was not getting anywhere. Sometimes I was besieged by doubts and I vainly attempted to shut off any thoughts of Enid. I thought of every conceivable method of combating my doubts. I tried to flood my mind with thoughts of Enid and my combined difficulties but that only made me more miserable. In doing that I had the vain hope that such an assault on my sensibilities might bludgeon me into insensitivity. I even considered trying to induce a nervous breakdown thereby leaving the subconscious to hopefully resolve the conflict in my mind. But in the end it seemed that I would have to try and resolve the conflict using the conscious rather than the unconscious part of the brain.

Then the answer came to me. I would take an overdose. I did not seriously think of killing myself, just of drawing attention to myself or at least finding a temporary release in drug induced oblivion. In the early part of November I went into Lampeter and bought a bottle of a hundred paracetamol tablets and a tube of the strongest aspirins on the market. These I placed in the cupboard in my room for I was not of the frame of mind to swallow them then.

Rag day came, but passed uneventfully except for one visit to Steve. I was feeling slightly jealous again and I complained to him of my sadness. He was dark-haired and thickset and was not as good looking as me but though I felt I had more sex appeal than him I envied him his stoicism. I had already started to confide in him about some of my difficulties and he told me that he himself had been rejected by a woman he loved but that the misery and the heartache had gone. He advised me to hold on saying that the sadness would eventually go. He also said that he had had a sex problem, that it had driven him "wild" at the time but that he had got over it. I believed my problems were more deep rooted than his and though Steve went further to understanding me than the others he didn't understand me fully. He assumed my feelings were due to having been rejected by Enid. He hadn't grasped the essence of the problem and I thought it wasn't his problem to bother about anyway. Problems were only the business of those paid to bother with them.

The next day I heard that Enid had spread my confidence about a nose correction. I was not particularly worried anymore by what people thought but nonetheless paid her a visit to establish the extent of the rumour. I also wanted an excuse for a final glimpse of her. I went up to her room at about three in the afternoon and to my surprise discovered that she was still in bed. I glanced at her guessing she must be completely naked. The sunlight was filtering through the closed curtains and in that light with the sheets draped over her, her luscious body outlined underneath, her blond hair spilling over the pillow, she looked like an Olympian Goddess. Her attitude was dismissive.

"I won't be a minute" I stammered looking at my watch and I asked her whom she had broken my confidence to.

"Only my two best friends " she snapped back.

I walked out of the room full of the knowledge that worshipping her would be my lot from now on and even that from a distance.

That Friday I attended the disco drunk with Nick. Nick's sister had come up for the evening and she and David were at the disco. I had a couple of dances but was not interested in anyone particularly on the dance floor and towards the end of the evening I left and made my way up to my room. David had left a little before me.

Once I had gained my room I opened the cupboard and took out the paracetamol tablets and the aspirins. I filled a glass and recklessly swallowed thirty paracetamol tablets in rapid succession. I did so with little feeling and little thought. Though not concerned at the possibility of dying I had not despaired of the possibilities of life and never envisaged myself dead.

After swallowing the tablets I waited for an effect. Nothing dramatic happened. In fact nothing happened. I had hoped Nick or someone might walk into my room that evening and find me in a comatose state. That I saw would never come about so I visited David who had a room in the Terrapins. I knocked on the door and he let me in. I couldn't bring myself to tell him I had taken an overdose. I felt nauseated and was sick on the floor. The spew seethed in a white puddle, the half-digested paracetamol tablets still evident in the pile. David did not twig that I had taken an overdose and such was his nature he did not even complain of the inconvenience. I still couldn't bring myself to admit the truth of the situation and after I had been sick I said "goodbye" and made my way back to Lloyd Thomas Hall.

Once there I was lost for what to do. I felt I couldn't leave the job half done and decided to go the whole way and try and induce a comatose state. I locked the door and swallowed most of the remaining paracetamol tablets followed by the aspirins. I secretly hoped that the cleaning lady would find me in the morning, forgetting she didn't come at weekends. I changed into my pyjamas and climbed into bed to await my release from my troubles. Soon I fell asleep.

Approximately three hours later I woke up feeling completely nauseated and was violently sick on the floor by my bed. Once I had started retching I couldn't stop. It went on and on. I had been sick before in my early experiments with alcohol but this was much worse. It seemed endless. It was as if I was sicking up the whole of my intestines. This was not attention seeking let alone peace of body and mind. It was punishment. I went on as such all night.

By the morning all that came out was a red slime. The floor by my bed was red. I got out of bed and staggered to the basin looking at my face in the mirror. My face was a deathly white. It was as if all the blood in my veins had been emptied onto the floor and I had a drink of water to try and clear my stomach and help restore the loss of liquid from my body. Afterwards I went back to bed again. Half an hour later I felt the need to be sick again and all the water I had drunk came up. I felt so physically ill at that moment I found that Enid and all my doubts had passed from my mind. All I thought about was the nausea.

By lunchtime I felt that I needed some sort of help to end the sickness which I thought was a slow way of dying; I also realised that it was now the weekend and that the cleaning woman wouldn't be coming. I unlocked the door of my room and crawled out onto the landing waiting for someone to come by. In due course someone did but I only asked him to get some milk, not a doctor. He did not seem concerned at the sight of me prostrate on all fours and returned with a carton of milk. I took it into my room and drank it. No sooner had I done so than I started to be sick again.

The second evening I felt so nauseated and weak I decided to ask for positive help. I crawled onto the landing. Someone came by and asked me if I had taken tablets. I said I had taken ten. He left and returned a little later to say that he had informed the porters in the porters lodge. I crawled back into my room and waited prostrate on my bed.

About half an hour later the nurse from the sanatorium knocked at my door. She said that an ambulance was coming and I packed certain items of clothing into a bag. I gathered up my shaving things, soap, shampoo and a pair of scissors and put them in a black shoulder bag and waited.

Finally the ambulance arrived. In a more hopeful frame of mind I put on my dressing gown and slippers and walked without aid down the stairs with my black shoulder bag to the ambulance. On the journey to "Carmarthen General Hospital" twenty miles away I started vomiting again directing the spew into a cardboard kidney dish held out to me by a sympathetic ambulance crewman and all that came out now was a frothing saliva. But as I drove through the interminable darkness to "Carmarthen General Hospital" I at least now had hope for I thought there I might find sympathy and understanding at last.

I sat down in hospital casualty which was almost empty and the few nurses who appeared left abruptly again without a word, almost as if they didn't deem me worthy of pity. Half an hour later a young doctor with a beard appeared.

"You bloody idiot" he said. It now seemed that I had not been correct about hospitals and that if I was hoping for sympathy I had come to the wrong place. "Come with me" said the doctor and I was led into another room and laid out on a couch. He roughly prodded me with his fingers. Then he left.

As I lay on the couch I thought: "If they can't show me sympathy they might as well try and understand me. They might as well try and get into my mind. They haven't even asked me how I feel." But at least I had escaped the dreaded stomach pump though only because I had vomited up so much it was probably deemed a waste of time.

After another half hour had passed a nurse came and escorted me to a ward. From what I could gather it was an emergency ward. I stepped into a bed with crisp, clean sheets. There I complained to a nurse of my nausea and I was given an injection to quell it. I was also put on a saline drip. After the nurse had left I sank into an uneasy sleep.

The following morning I had improved all-round and I had a better chance to take in my surroundings. There was a young lad who had taken an overdose after a rift with his girlfriend and there was a terminally ill leukaemia patient. The other patients were all in a bad way but were very friendly in contrast to the nurses who seemed to regard me as a nuisance for deliberately poisoning myself.

Later that day I was strong enough to sit up comfortably and to talk with ease. My drip was removed and then I was called into the interview room. Seated behind a desk was a doctor. I sat down in front of him and he started to question me. I had noted that that morning the young parasuicide had been discharged without having had a chance to air his problems and I did not want that state of affairs to arise again so I answered all the doctor's questions with that thought in mind. One was whether I had at any time been incoherent. I hadn't exactly been incoherent but I replied " yes" to the question to ensure I gained the attention I required. And that I achieved for the doctor ended up saying he would be putting me on another ward. I did not mind the idea although I didn't fully understand why I could not stay on the ward I was on.

I was pushed in a wheelchair down a corridor to the other ward by a male nurse. It gave me a feeling of importance to find myself being pushed in a wheelchair for up till now I had not been treated with any consideration. When I arrived at my new ward I was put in a section with two old men. Both were incontinent and that part of the ward reeked with excrement. They were suffering from senile dementia and I was put in a bed next to one.

I was asked to give in my scissors by another male nurse for my bag of things had been brought with me in the wheelchair. It was feared I might get hold of them and use them on myself. I was a little taken aback to think that the nurses thought I would do something so desperate for cutting myself was very far from my mind. But I handed them over without argument.

It was only after I had handed them over that I realised the ward I was on was a psychiatric unit and I suddenly felt angry. To have been put into a psychiatric unit I must have been deemed mad. So the doctor who had seen me had been a psychiatrist. I thought I was disturbed but I also thought there was a great difference between being disturbed and being mad. I had been rejected by society. I was viewed as a cripple. I was a "loony". It was a cruel awakening.

A little later the male nurse who had taken the scissors off me came back and started to crack jokes about the old man suffering from senile dementia in the bed next to mine. He also had a terminal intestinal condition and had tubes coming out of him with plastic bags attached. He had just relaxed his bowels again.

"Oh my God, you have shit yourself again" was the vein of the nurse's words. "You are a shit machine. That's all you are. A shit machine. Where's your brain? You haven't even got one."

My anger at what I was witnessing quickly became apparent and the nurse said: "Don't worry. He can't understand what I'm saying. He's demented."

Sadly that was how I was to sense people felt about me. The nurse it had transpired had wanted to go into the church but had gone into the nursing profession instead still treasuring the hope of one day being ordained. What he saw in the nursing profession had destroyed his faith.

When lunch came I found I was unable to eat. This was not appreciated by the staff. But I was given a glass of orange juice by the aforementioned nurse and that was all I really wanted anyway.

That afternoon a bloodtest was taken. I was grateful for the attention. It was the first I had had and I assumed it would be able to tell the doctors something.

However that afternoon I was still confused about the whole psychiatric set up and it appeared that only in medical wards did nurses wait upon patients. In psychiatric wards the patients were just left to get on with it. It was an approach I found hard to understand and to get used to. I also remained very insecure and I would have preferred to be at home where at least I would have had the love of my family. I was even dubious about whether I had achieved anything in coming into hospital.

The next day I saw three doctors. Even though most of the nurses did not display a great interest in my condition the doctors did a little all-round probing firstly on my physical state. I was asked how many tablets I had taken. I felt too silly to say I had taken over a hundred so again only admitted to having taken ten. I was informed paracetamol tablets attacked the liver and that death could be a delayed reaction to an overdose of them. All I was told was that the liver had remarkable powers of regeneration. I was asked to lie down on a couch and one doctor, the older and wiser of the three, probed the area round my liver. I was asked if I felt any pain. As I felt none I replied "no". That indicated I would survive as long as I liked. That concluded the interview.

The same day, John, Digby and Steve came to visit. I was pleased that they had made the effort even if I realised they did not really care. John and Steve were curious about the psychiatric set up. I revealed to them my initial anger at what I had seen but only Steve seemed to understand. To the others psychiatry was just another world, a world with many unpleasant aspects but a world that wasn't their concern. I spoke of the thing most on my mind, my thirst. I was eager for some pure fruit juice for I could not hold anything else down and I made the most of my visitors by sending them into town to buy some. They returned with the fruit juice and hastily left. They were the first and only visitors I was to receive. I saw I was probably becoming a burden to my friends and now that I was a psychiatric patient they would cease to believe in me.

On the third day I again saw the doctors. They saw each patient every weekday until the patient was fit to leave or otherwise be transferred. I appreciated the time given to me and the fact that the older doctor always spoke to me as if I was a colleague meant I didn't feel I was being looked down upon. But though Dr. E., my consultant, tried to be understanding the older doctor, the wise man, was the only one who contributed anything useful to the discussion. They were amazed at the result of the bloodtests taken on me which revealed I had taken considerably more than ten paracetamol tablets. I omitted to mention the underlying factor of my nose preoccupation but I spoke at length about Enid and bed which were more on my mind. I also told them of my tauntings and I spoke of her view that sex was the be all and end all of existence. The older doctor said that the appetite for food was stronger than the urge for sex but that did not help my thinking. I simply wanted to fit again and so face the world again. My ambition was to get married. This was a sign of my insecurity but also a concomitant of love. However when I looked round there were few people I wanted to marry.

Worse, always on my mind was the image of Enid, radiant and beautiful at her best and little offered itself as a substitute for that.

For the rest of the week I just lay in bed gathering strength. The unit was to open up a whole new world for me. I recall a man who used to walk past my section of the ward in his pyjamas and dressing gown calling for his dog. He was reliving his time in the Navy. One evening a man fell rigid on the floor by his bed in an epileptic seizure whilst the nurses held him down and tried to shove a pad between his teeth. From my point of view I began to feel that remaining in hospital was not likely to benefit me and after a week I asked if I could discharge myself. Dr. E. said that I was a voluntary patient and that I could go whenever I liked. Physically I had improved and I was able to eat again after the hammering the overdose had given my body. Mentally my self-confidence was still at a very low ebb even though it might have appeared that on the surface I had improved. I had told the nurses not to inform my parents of my O.D. and, determined not to go back to college that term, I asked my parents to come and take me home. They were quick to respond and after a detour to Lampeter where they picked up the remainder of my things they arrived at "Carmarthen General Hospital". I grabbed what personal effects I had and skipped out of the hospital with a great feeling of relief. Perhaps hospitals had the answers. Perhaps they didn't. But this hospital did not appear to have any.

I had had my first taste of hospitals. I had made my first cry for help. But those holidays I had to live with the fact that having sought help none had been forthcoming and I was now on my own. With this last avenue having turned out a dead end it was as if my problems had multiplied.

Those holidays I stayed with Mark Watts at Kentwell Hall in Suffolk for the weekend. He was helping towards the refurbishment of the vast Elizabethan mansion and there were plaster casts lying on the floor everywhere for the restoration of the tracery of the ceilings. As well as taking me for a guided tour of the rooms he showed me the grounds. I had written a letter to him at university and said I identified with the victim. It had been the first time I openly and consciously felt and stated that. It just intensified the mystery to him and he asked round trying to penetrate it. He knew of my scorn for the caveman mentality but I was clearly the loser. The weekend provided a welcome escape. I slept in a large four poster bed. But I was still unhappy underneath. My philosophy of turning the other cheek was deeply ingrained still though I didn't see its implications and still thought that by being physically perfect I would be happier again and fit in. And en route home I visited Dr. H.'s clinic in London.

Back at home I found myself retreating into my bedroom rarely going out and avoiding social activities. I felt sexually frozen and emotionally unresponsive to the people I encountered. I thought a Venus might provide the answer. But I steered clear of contact. The notion of free love and the liberated attitude of young people worried me. On the television downstairs I watched a boy meet girl story. Their relationship was founded on looks and a mutual skill in bed. It's basis was animal. It made me feel more inadequate, cut off and miserable. A whole new world had been closed to me, a world whose processes went to ensure the future of the human race.

One day a brief but powerful anger flared up in me. My confidence had been torn away and it was a rebound effect to what I was feeling. I went out into the garden, picked up a brick and banged a fence post. In my mind's eye was a picture of Enid's face and it was this or more precisely her nose that I was hitting though there was no intention or desire to actually hurt her. I felt the same thing for a minute or two the following day but otherwise remained just totally miserable.

The start of the new term came. Logically I should not have returned to university that term but I was determined not to sacrifice my university career because of a girl. But for Enid I felt I could have made a go of university. Now I was too miserable to do any justice to myself in my studies. However I did not harbour any resentment towards Enid. I had come to regard her purely with affection and the events of the previous term had by the end of the holidays gone to the back of my mind though I still had my preoccupations. Had I been perfectly confident about my looks I could have faced up to life. If I had been able to view Enid as good I could almost have faced up to life. If I could have overcome my problems I could have been a hero. None of these things was the case.

That first evening I sat in the union bar alongside Nick and David and managed to catch up on all that had happened in my absence. Nick was courting Lorna. Enid had acquired an additional boyfriend, an architect from London she said. David himself had made several more conquests and my other friends were making inroads in their relationships with women. Only I felt isolated and unhappy. No one held out hope and Nick, my best friend, was trying to avoid blaming Lorna for her part in my O.D. though I saw Lorna as a genuine lovely person. From what I could gather many people had thought it inadvisable for me to return to university that term and Enid had said as much to Nick. It was all in all an abysmal started but I determined to go to lectures the next day and to meet the challenges of the next few weeks. But that was being over-optimistic.

Then a little into the term, things reached a sudden crisis point. I was attending a Greek and Roman Civilisation lecture, attending in person rather than in spirit that is, when I saw Enid walking outside the window with her London boyfriend in the direction of the porters lodge. Never able to concentrate enough to take in but a small amount of what the lecturer was saying, I rose from my seat and walked hurriedly out of the room after Enid. I was curious to see her boyfriend from close up, to see what special qualities he had to command her respect. My manner of departure from the lecture was such that it provoked one female student to say:"Oh, he must be in love." By the time I had got out of the building Enid and her boyfriend had disappeared. I assumed that they must have entered the porters lodge near the main entrance so I had a peep inside. There I found her and her boyfriend perusing the notice board. I entered and walked over to the desk. I could hear Enid's dulcet tones clearly as she addressed him. I made some excuse to the porter on duty to the effect that I had locked myself out of my room. The porter, sensing my emotional state, launched into the attack: "What do you think you are doing losing your keys you bloody idiot?" Overcome I managed no more than the word "sorry". When I uttered the word my voice cracked. It was the first time this had happened. "I'll bring the key back as quickly as possible" I said with a hint of the same emotion. "You do that you bloody idiot" replied the porter. All the time Enid went on speaking as if nothing had happened. But I had been humiliated most terribly in front of her. I walked out of the porters lodge, head bowed, covered the distance to my room at an average pace and then returned to the porters lodge with the key. Enid and her boyfriend were gone. I was better able to collect my thoughts and spoke to the porter in more forthright tones. But I could not escape the thought of how I had humiliated myself in front of Enid and her boyfriend and left the porters lodge deeply concerned as to how I could make amends for my quaking voice that day.

That night the idea occurred to me to write a letter of explanation to Enid. I wanted to bolster up her image of me, that image that had been so badly dented by my being sent to a psychiatric unit, and thus to escape the shame I felt. I was not sure how much of the letter I meant but I at least wanted to set her straight on a couple of matters. I opened by exclaiming: "What illness is this?" I hoped that by putting her in the right and myself in the wrong her attitude might soften. I then said that just to glimpse her upset me, that the thought of her in bed with another man cut me to the quick and the sight of her with another man drove me wild. I said I was only deeply attracted to one in forty women. I was trying to make her see the truth of my love for her and in turn trying to make her value it. I then started to apologise again to appease her. I said that the effect she usually had on me was to make me sad, not anger me. I signed off with the words: "Goodbye little girl, Andrew" and put the letter in her pigeonhole.

The next day I told John of my letter and the next evening as we sat drinking our pints in the bar alongside two other girls, friends of both Steve and Enid, Enid happened to come by. I observed her out of the corner of my eye and to my utter amazement she did not just continue on her journey but came and sat down two places to my right. I dared not look at her, but I looked down at my lap. However I sensed her presence there. She only remained seated for a minute or two before getting up and walking out of the union bar. I glimpsed her departing face and saw that it was sad. She disappeared up the union building stairs on the way to her room and John said afterwards that he saw her wipe a tear from her eye as she left us. One of the two girls got up as well and followed after her. John said to me: "Well, she must like you." I was relieved just to be seen as human again. I thought it was the end of her silly games. The worst thing in the end to face was being treated like a disease and she seemed to have shown she had a conscience, that she was at least human and that I was human.

The next day and the day after that I saw her round the university but she did not acknowledge me again. She had made her gesture. Now she had full control of her emotions again and I was confronted by the same iron hard Enid I had known before. Her London boyfriend also still appeared and I could not fail to see them walk past my window in Lloyd Thomas Hall so I decided to move to the Terrapins at the other end of the campus. The room I was given was opposite David's and he helped in the arrangements. I hoped that in the Terrapins I would be out of her way.

A few days later I went to the union bar with a gang of friends and got drunk on cider. The gang included amongst others, Mark, Richard and Tony. Mark had big nostrils. As the gang was composed of largely good looking individuals it was as a whole very conscious of how people looked and Mark, because of his big nostrils, had difficulty in getting accepted by the gang. But he was tall and confident, he had had a certain amount of sexual experience and understood the ways of the world and was therefore partially accepted. Richard on the other hand, despite his gentle disposition and lack of assertiveness had an essentially delicate classical appearance which made him acceptable to the gang. Tony was a friend of David's and for that reason became involved with the group. He was well built and regular featured. Nick always thought of me as better looking than Tony though Tony had a better nose and a thicker set body. I too was easily accepted. The gang went to discos, to cafes in Lampeter and to the refectory and that night was drinking alcohol and planning to go to the disco in the Arts building. At the disco I asked a girl to dance. In the coloured light of the dance hall she looked attractive. I saw her a day or two later when a fault became apparent though she seemed a nice girl. And towards the end of the evening the itch to see Enid became too great to withstand.

David had left the disco earlier and at about half past ten I walked back to the Terrapins and ambled into David's room.

"I'm going to commit suicide " I said. He didn't believe me and I didn't believe myself but I was determined to do something dramatic. David just sat there his normal equable but tired self. As if in desperation at finding such a lack of recognition at my plight I walked out of his room up to Enid's door. I hoped that her reaction to me would in some way influence my feelings, either to reassure me or to drive me to deeper despair and so prompt a suicide attempt. She was usually up at this hour so I did not think it an untimely moment to visit her. I knocked on the door of her room and waited for her to open it. She was rather a long time about it and in an effort to look casual I turned round so that my back faced the door stuffing my hands in my pockets. She did eventually open the door but on noticing me there she banged it shut again. I turned round but only succeeded in catching a quick glimpse of her. I grabbed hold of the doorknob and pushed it; the door remained firmly shut. Even now I realised she did not trust me. I stood for a couple of minutes outside her room to collect myself then left and made my way back to the Terrapins.

Back in my room, my feelings still of sadness, I made my way to the dressing table, took a new razor blade from the top drawer with the idea of cutting my wrists, and walked into the washroom. I filled a basin with piping hot water and placed my right hand and wrist in the water. I took a firm grip of the razor blade, immersed it in the water and scratched the under part of my right wrist. The incision was not deep enough to draw much blood. I decided to cut the other wrist instead and dipped my left arm in the water and attempted to slice the veins under my left wrist holding the blade with my right hand. There was still only a drop of blood so I steeled myself to cut a little deeper in the same place. After that the blood poured out. Although I had often thought of the Ancient Romans who used this method for committing suicide and I had got the idea of cutting my wrists from them I still did not have it in mind to kill myself. What I was doing was purely and simply another cry for help. Blood was something I believed people would react to and I hoped the blood that I drew would draw attention to myself. It would be an outward manifestation of my inward pain. So with hope of a reaction from David I walked into his room. David looked up from his bed where he was sitting and noticed the blood.

"Oh my God" he exclaimed. "I had no idea. Christ, what you must have been feeling."

I sat down in his chair and he got up from the bed, knelt down beside me and put his arms round me. I felt his warmth flood through me displacing much of the sadness. He had shown true compassion, the love that Christ had exhibited for mankind. It was a side of human beings that I hardly ever saw. Enid had shown a tiny hint of it if in her case it had been mixed with guilt and both feelings she had deliberately shut out for they did not conform to her idea of the world. But David was largely uncorrupted by the world and at that moment pure goodness flowed from his heart. Experience can poison goodness, but he had retained some of his childhood innocence and that was what I was seeking to find in people. That was the first step in getting out of people the advice and help I required. I felt that if I could find where there was goodness in the world there would be some hope for me. If people were all as egocentric as Enid then there would be no hope for me. But David had displayed the warmth of goodness. Comfortably rejuvenated I got up.

"I think I'll go to bed now" I said and returned to my room.

That same night, so I discovered later, David, unable to keep his secret to himself, went and informed Nick of what had happened and the following morning he and Nick came round to my room. They waited for me to dress and then all three of us went to the bus stop and waited for the bus to Carmarthen where I wanted my wrists seen to; of course it was my mind I really wanted seen to. At the bus stop I told Nick and David not to tell John of my so-called suicide attempt. The reason for this was that I was frightened of being viewed as an object of contempt. I knew that John would only see it as a mark of failure and therefore worthy of contempt. I wanted help, not the contempt of people. David and Nick were as many confidantes as I needed. In Carmarthen we walked to the outpatients department of the general hospital. A doctor came and spoke to us and I showed him my wrists. He led me into a busy "surgery" and made me sit down. He said giving me an anaesthetic would hurt me more than just stitching me up. Then he took hold of my wrist and started to stitch as if it was the cuff of a shirt. The pain was localised but sharp and though I succeeded in keeping my wrist relaxed I writhed internally and gritted my teeth. Fortunately it was a short operation and with a great sense of relief I saw the needle pass out of my skin for the last time. The stitches were then covered up.

Sadly I had been in too much pain to ask the questions I wanted to ask and the doctor had not begun to probe my psyche. However after the stitching he did go and ask David and Nick if they thought I needed psychiatric help. They both said "no". As we were leaving the hospital Nick informed me of what the doctor had asked and they had answered. I appreciated their faith in me but I realised that my "suicide attempt" had in the end achieved little. I was still burdened with my troubles and I had not been offered the chance of assistance. I was beginning to feel that there was goodness in the world but I could not depend on people like David.

I did however have a rather unexpected surprise that very same day when I discovered a note in my pigeonhole from Enid. It went as follows:

"Dear Andrew, I apologise for my abrupt refusal to see you last night. You are welcome to come to tea tomorrow at three o'clock. It would be nice if you could make it."

The note was written on a scruffy bit of paper torn from an exercise book but it was the sentiments it appeared to express that mattered to me, not the paper. I showed it to John who commented: "Well she must like you."

I took up Enid's invitation to come to tea with her in her room full of hopes for a better world. It was as agreed three o'clock and a teapot, milk jug, and tea cups and saucers were laid on a table. Enid's crochet rug was still on her bed and the whole room was meticulously clean and tidy. Enid was wearing a pair of jeans that exaggerated the size of her thighs but was otherwise very pretty even if I was no longer quite so enthralled by the magic of her room.

She started by saying that she was in the middle of an essay so when I sat down I resolved not to remain seated long. I had not myself felt that I had pestered her up till now and was not going to start pestering her at this stage.

She poured out the tea then came forth with one piece of advice: "Take up rugby." I thought that was a hint at developing my body, increasing my aggressiveness and developing stamina. If I couldn't bring up my rating by improving my nose I could turn myself into a he-man body wise. But as I did not consciously think of brutishness in sexual relations I was loath to think of myself as a rugby playing lover.

I gulped down my cup of tea then said: "Well, I will let you get on with your essay" and left. I left with the knowledge that whatever Enid had to say about my problem existing purely in my head as she had once said, I still had to get over the attitude of certain women, particularly pretty ones which was such that they were only able to respond to beautiful looks or some indeterminate notion of the perfect body. But I did leave Enid's room with the belief that perhaps good might dominate over bad after all for she had at least appeared good, kind and understanding. I was sorry to leave her. It almost made me cry tearing myself away from such gracefulness, gentleness and good looks. But the main thing was my opinion of her moral worth had improved.

Afterwards I went on to tell my friends how pleasant she had seemed. I even said that I must have been mistaken about her, that she was after all a good, honest and genuine person. My friends all nodded their heads in accord. They went on to say that I had seen the light. What I couldn't have known was that the meeting had in fact been set up by John and Digby who had been informed I had cut my wrists and that Enid had been very reluctant to it. The only good thing was that I no longer had the need to see or call on Enid again.

Amazingly I didn't find lectures so daunting after that and I made a strong effort to attend. It was almost as if I was an ordinary person again just suffering the pangs of unrequited love. It is possible to study under such a burden. Only when you feel worthless and without hope of good that all incentive goes and effort seems pointless. To look outwards, to meet the challenges posed by life, to show people that you are a force in the world should ensure that people respect you. I knew that I could not depend on the world being generally good and kind but this illusion of good on the part of Enid nonetheless buoyed me.

The scratches to my wrists soon healed up and in a better frame of mind I went to see my G.P. to have the stitches removed. It was evening and outside surgery hours so I had to go to his home in Lampeter. Nick accompanied me to lend me moral support. We knocked on the door and he let us into the hall. The G.P., whom I had never met before, turned out to be a very pleasant, understanding, warmhearted individual and even instanced an episode in his life when he had been let down by a girl so as to prove to me I was not alone in my discomforture.

"You will look back on this one day and think what a fool you were" he said of my scratched wrists.

I knew that had it been a question of a simple broken heart there would have been no problem. I did not mention my ongoing sadness but my G.P. asked me to see him the next day to discuss my troubles and of course to remove the stitches. He didn't have the required equipment at home for the job. As well as being encouraging, friendly and open he issued a warning. He said that a female patient he had had cut her wrists thirty times achieving nothing and that by cutting my wrists I could sever the tendons and nerves and end up limp-wristed.

The next day came and I waited my turn in the queue to see the G.P. and after a few minutes was called into the surgery. The G.P. was his same friendly self and I felt I could open out. But beyond a few encouraging words he did not have anything constructive to say. He went onto remove the stitches which fortunately proved to be a painless business. As advice did not seem to be the whole answer he prescribed anti-depressants and we both hoped that these would be the complete answer. I left the surgery in a more optimistic frame of mind.

I then went to the Chemist in Lampeter, acquiring the prescribed tablets which I looked upon as "happiness pills" and over the next few days attempted to see if pills, as claimed, could promote true happiness. The anti-depressants prescribed had been highly recommended in medical journals but the effect they had on me was to make me irritable, not happy. I couldn't honestly claim any good results. At Lancaster University I had read some graffiti on the wall of Fylde college toilets: "Don't adjust your brain. Reality is at fault." All pills could do were to interfere with your response to reality. And after five days I put the pills aside so that if ever I should feel miserable again I could take them all in one go and so blot out reality.

After all that had happened I was naturally still interested in my nose, the thing I regarded as the underlying cause of my unhappiness, the thing that had made me so vulnerable to the things Enid had said and done. In fact I thought of myself as something of a connoisseur on noses and I started to discuss noses with a few of my friends. I was still confident enough not to allow my concern over my nose to make me open to attack or to excite the contempt of my friends. But my nose and noses generally became the chief topic of conversation. Mark's nose came under attack and the inevitable parallels were drawn between it and the nose of a mask of a gorilla on the wall of Nick's room. Nick was cruel about Mark's nose but was kind about mine and many hours were wasted in idle comparison of noses. The noses were mostly good. Nick's nose had a hint of Charlton Heston's nose. My nose, though far from perfect, was considered superior to Lee Major's nose. The other noses were all considered appropriate for any world renowned sex symbol. Nick, Mark and I then went on to decide upon what was the perfect Caucasian nose. We eventually agreed upon certain principles determining this and it was agreed my nose could be improved in the interests of deification. As our other features were adequate our discussions were usually confined to noses.

Then I discovered what seemed to be the answer to the problem with my nose and thus the complete answer to my problems. Dr. H. had taken away its length thus destroying its slimness and I came to believe that the answer lay in lengthening it, something I thought was surgically possible. Once I thought I could look upon imperfection as a temporary matter I experienced a psychological transformation. My sadness completely left me and if at first I had been genuinely in love with Enid it was only my own insecurity that had led me to continue to think of her and that same insecurity had generated in me feelings that masked as love. Aesthetics I had come to regard as basic. In order to master the basics of life I had to have my aesthetic sense satisfied. As my aesthetic sense stood to be satisfied by surgery it was as if all my cares had developed wings and flown.

I had arranged for the correction to my nose to take place at the end of term at Dr. H.'s clinic and went on to finalise the arrangements full of hope of success. I wrote to my father and told him of my plans and he wrote back to say that my nose had already lost its slimness and advised me against the idea. I was confident that if Dr. H. would only listen to me I would be all right.

At the end of term Nick saw me off on the coach and I departed with one suitcase on my fateful journey to London. I spent one night with Jerome then I went to the clinic. On my arrival there the auburn-haired nurse let me into the waiting room. The clinic was becoming very familiar to me and I had that same feeling of anticipation that my arrival there always gave me. I sat down in a velvet armchair with a magazine. A few minutes later Dr. H. entered and I stood up and attempted to explain what I wanted. With an unsure look on his face he walked out of the room. Soon afterwards the auburn-haired nurse returned.

"Noses can become an obsession" she said.

Dr. H. reappeared and together he and the nurse scrutinised me. "It does look slightly bulbous" the nurse commented of my nose.

The deviated septum wasn't observed but I was relieved that a major area of complaint had been noticed. Dr. H. saw things differently.

"You should have let me fracture the bone" he said looking at the bridge. "I could have done things with the nose then."

He took one more look and walked out of the room. I again became worried. I desperately tried to explain to the nurse what I wanted done.

"Dr. H. is the expert" she replied very simply. "Let him do what he thinks best."

She left the room and I was left on my own to ponder the matter. I wondered where the grey-haired nurse was. I hadn't seen her about and considered the possibility that she might have felt that I felt that I had been let down by her and thus asked not to be present. Dr. H. undoubtedly had his successes but I clearly wasn't one of them and she appreciated that.

The auburn-haired nurse reappeared and gave me a sedative. Ten minutes later she led me to the operating room. I was completely unprepared and full of doubts about the possible outcome.

I lay down on the operating table. My face met the full glare of the light and Dr. H. started on part two of his original plan. It was a painless business this time. Two hours of painless destruction. Afterwards Dr. H. said: "You will have all the girls after you" as if that was my real ambition. It was not and I was in two minds whether to believe him. I got off the table and rested in a chair for an hour in the upstairs room after which time Dr. H. ordered a taxi and together we drove to the accommodation address.

When I entered the flat I discovered that there had only been one other nasal refinement, namely of a person who had backed out the previous year and he and I were the only two patients in the flat. Obviously " difficult " patients were dealt with separately from the rest. I was given a room of my own to sleep in and I was very much on my own for Dr. H., who was staying over night, spent most of his time with the other patient. My room had two beds and a basin and a mirror above it. The bedroom was very feminine and was obviously designed for female patients, but was comfortable and I did not complain. By the side of each bed was a little bedside table and each table was piled high with women's magazines. I was very nervous and worried but could do little to help the situation and just lay on my bed and stared at the ceiling ignoring the reading matter. That evening Dr. H. briefly looked into my room.

"You funny boy " he said and walked out again.

The next day my nervousness increased. Because of the dressing and "brace" round my nose I could only imagine what it looked like but I was even more dubious about what the results would be. By the second night I was so overcome by curiosity I got out of bed, switched on the light and went over to the mirror. I removed the brace, carefully loosened the dressing and slipped it off. I was horrified. All shape seemed to be lost and the result was the opposite of what I had wanted or planned. I replaced the dressing and brace and went back to bed in a state of shock. I succeeded in going back to sleep that night but only with difficulty.

The next morning my eyes wandered over to the magazines next to my bed. I picked up one and anxiously started to look through it pausing at all the advertisement pages to examine the features of the male models. I still could not find a nose that resembled mine. That morning I expressed my fears to Dr. H.. He remained his normal self but did not approve of my removing the covering. "Wait for the swelling to go down" he advised. Going on the last effort the change would only be slight even then.

My three days were up and I walked back to the clinic with Dr. H. for the removal of the dressings. I hardly looked at the mirrors in the clinic after they had been removed. It was as if I didn't want to see the truth. I left for the underground with a terrible feeling of loss. On the underground people gave me strange glances. I was bruised and swollen and boarding the Devon train at Waterloo I felt even more self-conscious and different than after part one. A view of myself in the Gentlemans revealed not only a worse but a more feminine appearance.

At Honiton I detrained and telephoned for my mother. She picked me up in the car and drove me home. I was now truly miserable. The floodgates of my emotions were opening and it was a struggle holding back the tears. I had set about climbing the one high peak of a lifetime and had lost my footing. At home I deposited my suitcases in the hall and did a tour of all the mirrors in the house. None of the reflections were of comfort. I was ugly or if not that ordinary. I felt as if I had been disfigured. I felt totally ruined.

That afternoon I went for a drive with my sister in her Mini. She had plenty of boyfriends and though she was not perfect she made do. She did not go to the lengths that I did to achieve the ultimate, whatever that might be. Yet she was able to sympathise with me.

We drove to Hembury fort, a local beauty spot. The area was thickly wooded and the spring leaves had yet to unfold on the trees. We got out of the car and walked for a bit. The dead leaves left over from the previous autumn still lay on the ground in a partial state of decay and I crunched them underfoot. I didn't have it in me to walk far and my sister and I shortly returned to the car. On the way home I started to weep. At home I went up to my bedroom. I sat down on the floor in a state of abject despair. There I began to weep even more. I had never been so wretched in my life. It was as if all my hopes had come to nought, my dream ruined. I had not thought about Enid once in the last four days. I was purely concerned with the centre of my face, my nose. I momentarily thought of a shotgun as a means of suicide. That was the true mark of the pain I was in. The grief was so deep I felt myself briefly pass out.

When I recovered my sister and mother were next to me holding me. My father was out on parish business and thus missed the drama, but my mother and sister who had been downstairs had been attracted by the sounds I was making and had come upstairs to see what the matter was. I felt I urgently needed help and said:

"I want to go to a hospital."

Though hospitals had not helped me before I hoped they might help me now. My mother helped me onto the bed and she and my sister comforted me. I knew I had deliberately let myself go. It was the first time I had let myself go. Now I resolved not to allow that to happen again and for the remainder of the afternoon and for the duration of the evening I kept a hold of myself as best I could. I also always insisted on having someone next to me for it reassured me and for the first time in my life I did not feel entirely in control. My mother said she would take me to the doctor.

That evening I stood in front of the mirror in my room and played about with the ghastly mess that had once been a nose. I had despaired of the idea of a normal life, of being happy. I had prepared myself to exist only partially, to being able to indulge only half the senses, to being a robot that just works and refuels. Then as I smoothed over the bridge with my fingers the nose started to subside and settle. The nose had taken on a new shape. It had assumed some sort of form out of the formlessness. I was still not happy, the refinement had been retrogressive. But I was better able to tolerate it now.

The next day I was taken to see the family G.P.. I spoke to him in his surgery alone and told him I was suffering from depression. He was reluctant to get involved and simply said: "See your doctor back at university." Up till now none of the doctors had any helpful advice to give. Psychiatry it seemed was still in the dark ages. As far as psychiatry was concerned there was no quick answer. I felt truly let down.

But those holidays I did manage to do some work for my English literature syllabus writing an essay on St. Mawr by D.H. Lawrence. Though I had lost most of my motivation I nevertheless strove towards the goal of academic success. I was determined not to let the world and its barbs prevent me from obtaining the qualifications necessary to get on in life. All I had left was the hope of achieving respectability in a career. Yet if drudgery was all that was left for me I might as well make a pleasure of it. Even so it seemed that everything went together. The need for personal fulfilment and the need for fulfilment career-wise were part of a joint motivation with me. Some could divorce the two or make up for one with the other, but I came to believe I could only achieve fulfilment in one if I achieved fulfilment in the other.

Oneday those holidays I went to the nearby city of Exeter with my father, mother and sister, and being amongst crowds again made me more self-conscious. I was worried that I was no longer noticed. After we had done our required shopping we went to a Wimpey bar for a cup of coffee. I looked around at the customers seated at the other tables and the waitresses who carried on as if I didn't exist, as if I was a non-person. I feared being insignificant. I mentioned this to my father:

"I can't understand why you should continue to worry about your nose" he replied. "Look at my nose and I don't worry about it." My father had a rather long and ugly nose. I was now faced with the fact that no-one could truly understand my plight or dependency. It was like trying to adapt to being a nonentity. It was a difficult change to make. People often dictated what I should feel and I was always being told I should be this or I should be that. I was never told quite how I could change from being what I was. It was almost a relief to get back to the country that day for being buried alive in the countryside at least obscured the fact that I was now a nonentity.

Near the end of the holidays I went up to London to see Dr. H. and I stayed the night with Jerome in his flat. Jerome was staunchly supportive and made me almost believe there was such a thing as true friendship. Despite his encouragement I felt no better. I had cut some pictures of Tom Jones out of a magazine. He had had his face remodelled in the cause of megastardom though a sex symbol before. I laid them out on the carpet in the lounge and examined them. Tom Jones' new nose, though small, had shape. A critical view of my nose was that it was too small, too short, stuck out slightly and was rounded at the tip. I was by no means a gargoyle. I did not think I would scare away young children or that I would be mocked or laughed at. Externally I had not suffered like a third degree burns victim. But form and proportion had been lost. (In fact it wouldn't have taken much to make the nose as good as Tom Jones' nose but I had no idea how then.)

The following morning Jerome went off to work and I to Dr. H.'s clinic. It was he who let me in and there were no nurses present. He took me upstairs and walked around me observing me from every angle.

"It will turn out a nice nose" he said.

Dr. H. was the psychologist supreme. It was his hope that in time I would get used to my changed face and so would be able to accept it. But it seemed whether I accepted my changed face depended on whether I would be accepted with it. I left the clinic with little faith left in anyone.

I had two more nights before the actual start of term and the next day I travelled to Carmarthen directly from London. Nick and his mother picked me up near the coach station and I went to spend the night at the family home, Towy castle, built on the sight of the original castle with a lovely view over a loop in the river Towy. That afternoon Nick showed me the house, the garden and the shrubbery. The all-round beauty acted as a tonic on my tortured nerves.

The next day I had to return to college and Nick's mother drove us there. It was a worrying moment for me for all the students would be returning that day. They, unlike Nick's parents, would be in a position to see a change in my appearance having seen me before and I had again to consider how the other students might react. On our arrival I left Nick and his parents and went off on my own wondering aimlessly about the university. I was still distraught and thought continuously: "Oh, can my face be changed back to how it was originally?" I kept noticing my reflection in plain glass. The shadow accentuated my faults and the only way to settle myself down then was to go and look at my reflection in an ordinary mirror as in white light it wouldn't look quite so bad even if I still saw how it fell short of perfection. When I strolled into the union bar that evening dressed in my suit for an official dinner and no one looked up at me, I realised the truth of the matter; even in my navy blue suit I was not striking anymore. When it came to going to the dinner I just could not face it and wandered back to the Terrapins alone.

When lectures started the next day I attended and did my level best to concentrate, mostly unsuccessfully. I recalled my last weeks at Lancaster University when my inability to concentrate had amongst other things led to my decision to leave. I wondered if leaving was a sign of cowardice. I was always unearthing reasons for running away from life. If I was to run now I would be trying to run away from the inescapable, my face. Logic said I should try and work for status and a career. I should try and avoid becoming an all-round failure, the sort that the gang occasionally made fun of. But what I was suffering from now seemed to me far worse than unrequited love. It was a lifelong disappointment. I resolved just to sit it out and try and face up to things as best I could.

Sadly, that was not to be so easy as was apparent two days after the start of term when I bumped into Enid. I was walking down a street in Lampeter with three or four friends. Then there she was some thirty yards away. She had on tight blue corduroys and an attractive white jumper and looked very pretty. At the sight of her I experienced a painful stab in the heart. I had not noticed her in the refectory and had almost forgotten about her. Now I had been reminded of her beauty. I turned and led my friends off in another direction.

By the end of the first week the idea of suicide had begun to form in my mind though again I was not seriously thinking about it. I did not know whom I could turn to for help. No one showed the slightest interest in my plight. Ernest Hemingway had shot himself it had been said because he was impotent. Even if I did not have the courage and will to actually commit suicide it did give me comfort to think that there was a way out in oblivion and my mind turned back to guns.

So about seven days after the beginning of term I went into a gunshop in Lampeter and examined the guns stacked in the glass case. I looked obviously miserable and was given a quizzical look by the assistant and told I would have to get a shotgun certificate if I wanted to buy one. I left a little disappointed that acquiring guns was not such an easy thing to do after all.

A day or two later I heard that Digby had a gun he wanted to sell. I visited him in his room in the Terrapins to enquire about it. He produced the gun, a single barrelled shotgun, for me to see. I handled it relieved that in this instrument of destruction I had hope of oblivion. Digby then said that Tony was also interested in buying it. I left the room without it.

That same day I decided to get a form for a shotgun certificate and then discussed the matter of obtaining a shotgun with John and Steve. They knew I was miserable but did nothing to dissuade me from getting the gun. Indeed they gave me some advice on how to fill out the form. In getting a reference I said it was for pheasant shooting.

A day or two later, still miserable, I paid a return visit to the gunshop and obtained a pamphlet of other guns as I thought a shotgun was a bit awkward and unwieldy as a method of self-destruction. I went to Tony's room to discuss the various guns with him as he had some knowledge of guns. Richard appeared on the scene and we three spread the pamphlet out on Tony's desk and discussed the different guns. I didn't come to any conclusions. I was just considering possible ways out and there was nothing sinister in it at all.

As I was not at all sure that shooting myself would be the best way out I still kept open the option of another nasal refinement and I hunted around for addresses of clinics in the popular journals. One address kept recurring and I visited the clinic in London but decided not to bother.

I received a letter to say my application form for a shotgun certificate had been turned down. I later found out that a policeman had visited my parents and asked them if they thought I should be granted one. They had replied: "Definitely not." I wondered what options were still open to me.

I might have been able to continue adequately with my university life but for one more awful blow. It was when Nick informed me, as we were sitting in his room, that the meeting I had with Enid the previous term immediately after scratching my wrists, had after all been set up by John and Digby, the two people I had asked should not be told about it. I made my way up to John's room and he told me that at his meeting with Enid she had tried to make out I was just "sick in mind" and that I wasn't to be looked upon as a normal person. John had embarrassingly answered that the problem might have been due to my doubts about bed. Enid had then claimed that my relationship with her was purely "a figment" of my "imagination" thus trying to clear herself. John had replied over dramatically: "It's a matter of life and death" and it was only with considerable reluctance that she had written the note inviting me to tea. I could understand that she might have been embarrassed to be linked with me at that stage but that she should lie so, that she should be so unconcerned that my life had to all appearances been in the balance, that she should turn me into a laughing stock in the eyes of all my friends at such a critical moment, was just too bitter a pill to swallow. I was now looked upon as a lunatic, not a normal human being anymore. At that moment I thought Enid could only be evil. Having made my shock known to John I returned to the Terrapins and walked into David's room. I said in an angry tone of voice: "This is the last straw."

My feelings of anger, frustration and betrayal were aggravated by my loss of confidence over the retrogressive nasal refinement the previous holidays and as a way of venting them I decided to write a letter to Enid. I went and sat down at the desk in my room and put pen to paper. I said that she had destroyed everything I believed in and that I had nothing to live for now telling her to get out of my life. Before putting the letter her pigeonhole I showed it to John who thought it justifiable.

That evening I was still slightly fuming so went and got drunk on four pints of cider. With that the remainder of my inhibitions fell away. I went and picked up a brick outside John Richards Hall that was still in the process of being constructed and hit a plank with it. I then carried the brick and the plank up to John's room and showed him the dent.I don't recall actually beating a plank. I wanted him to see how wronged I had been as I felt especially humiliated in front of him. Later I placed a brick from the building site in my black shoulder bag carrying it to the union bar. I then took it up to Enid's room in the bag with a far-off idea of tapping her on the nose with it. In actual fact it was virtually inconceivable that I would have used it as the idea was impracticable and my feelings were never more than a simple desire to punch her on the nose though she had made me feel so weak and inadequate that I believed a bare fist would not have remotely hurt her. Anyway she was out. I carried the brick to Mark's room and showed it to Mark indicating I would like to break Enid's nose with it. It was again my way of trying to get across the injustice I had suffered. But I threw the brick away afterwards. I returned to Tony's room where the core of my friends had gathered. It was then that I glimpsed a shotgun propped up in the corner of the room. It was the same shotgun that Digby had been wanting to sell to Tony. A little later, in a desperate attempt to make my friends understand I picked up the shotgun. Digby was present and had been treating me as the liar rather than Enid, the real liar.In frustration I probably said I could blast her but in fact I never actually wanted to hurt Enid, just get the truth across. My two so-called suicide attempts weren't serious and my indignation was in equal measure to my hurt which meant I never wanted to seriously hurt Enid. After Digby had left I carried the gun outside a few yards wrapped in a blanket, not because I had any plans to do anything but to try and get my friends to take me seriously. My life had been turned into a joke. I wanted to win back respect and credibility. I then went to the union bar and got David. And appreciating that I was only making myself look ridiculous I retrieved the gun in its blanket and handed it to him. In a pub in Lampeter the idea of smearing excrement in Enid's room was raised with John and Digby and others volunteering to contribute turds but we were not being totally serious and I was just pleased now it had been acknowledged I had been wronged. That helped my state of mind considerably.

Although I popped a note into Enid's pigeonhole a couple of days later, a pleasant note, expressing my embarrassment at the lack of objectivity in my letter, I knew she remained a dangerous proposition. I later discovered she had even been trying to get me charged with a criminal offence because of the letter I had sent her though I had avoided being threatening in it and it in fact contained the truth.

I had felt betrayed and angry over my discovery of the unfortunate events subsequent to my scratching my wrists. But my feelings of sadness soon asserted themselves over everything. More than once I felt the need to go and cry and once left Nick's room where some of my friends were congregated locking myself in the toilet. I was again nervous of being mocked in my despair and in private I let the tears flow. I found myself on my knees reduced to that posture I didn't know how. In a sense I was kneeling to Enid. I recalled that in the first term I had thought of her as a kind of goddess but with the needs and aspirations of a fallen woman. If she had been something distant and ethereal I could have coped with her. I could have loved and honoured her in a spiritual way. The fact that she was a worldly person who told lies, fornicated and hated made her all the more difficult to cope with.

From now on the pressures I was to come under were of a small but cumulative nature. They did not in themselves affect me too much but were indicative of my all-round decline.

The first of these small pressures occurred when Nick said in Tony's room that Enid had finally decided to get married and in the Catholic church. Because of her contempt for religion I thought it hypocritical and it was as if the worldly values embraced by her were by some ironic twist to receive the blessing of the church. On hearing the news I felt the tears rush to my eyes.

It was also about this time that my friends started to rag me about my nose particularly over the meal table. I had cut off my nose to spite my face was their attitude. They said my face was fat. It was the thing to be a stud. My comments to Nick indicated I wasn't. Such talk drew guffaws of laughter. I had used the term aardvark, an animal with a long proboscis. They called me aardvark except that rather than being too long my complaint was that my nose was too short. But in fact the teasing was very gentle. I later joked about starting off a stud farm for my friends where they could breed to their hearts content. And I was aware that something like an obsession over a nose could excite laughter and with all the lies about me how else could my friends react?

The morning after the first bout of ragging Nick spoke to me in the corridor outside the door of his room in Lloyd Thomas Hall:

"You know Andrew, if you insist on going on about your nose so much people are bound to take the Mickey out of you." I stuck by my friends not only because I appreciated this but because I could not exist on my own, particularly at this critical time. I also felt the need to talk about what was troubling me and I couldn't just sit there and pour out all my woes to a complete stranger. My friends were mostly very pleasant, agreeable and amusing and were only rarely discouraging or defamatory. Otherwise I would have had nothing more to do with them. It was only as a gang that they teased me as indeed they teased Mark.

The one bright occurrence was that Julie, who had been hostile to me in the first term, had now observed another side to my nature that she liked and even suggested I study up in her room if I thought that would help me concentrate. She liked me quiet and I was fairly withdrawn now. The offer I declined.

And with no hope of an answer to the problems that so weighed me down I lapsed into maudlin preoccupations with looks, Enid and physical relationships. One day I ambled out of the university campus turning right. I would often go for walks to get away from things. I walked into a football field adjacent, lay down on the grassy verge and with tears in my eyes thought about Enid and her concept of heaven. It lay in the physical, in the sexual act. Going on her words to me I thought about her being satisfied by a big burly virile handsome lover with bedsprings creaking and bodies thrashing about. Then I thought of myself. My bed was the long crisp grass, the only pleasure I enjoyed was self-pity.

But it was not all a question of maudlin preoccupations. Nick and I went out onto the tennis courts. It was a warm summer's day and it was good getting some fresh air and exercise. We hit the ball back and forth to one another over the net, one of several long rallies. Nick noted my game. I had mastered the basics of stroke play though normally he did not have a player competent enough to give him a decent game. I did not see myself as being of more than average club standard.

Enid unfortunately still had her claws in me playing with me like a cat with a mouse. The idea of having someone churned up emotionally over her appealed to her. One day I was in Steve's room when he said: "She's walking all over you." He had been doing some scouting around and repeated someone else's words: "She's a bunch of razor blades." Another person had said she had "a definitely evil streak" and that she was "dangerous". I assumed that other people like me must have witnessed the darker side of her personality. I was pleased it was acknowledged that she did have this darker side to her personality. But acknowledgement of that fact changed nothing. My friends now respected me just as little and Enid remained just as respected. Very little bad was said about her unless it reflected badly on me as well.

I was speaking to Nick. He said that Enid had been a nurse in a mental hospital. Did that explain it? I surmised that it was in a mental hospital that she learnt all about the mechanics of the human mind and perfected her unprecedented talent for personal manipulation, confirmed her belief that there was no such thing as God, that heaven was just an idea invented to give people like me hope and that there was no such thing as a moral power outside of ourselves.

I began to contemplate changing my mental outlook. I could not concede that there was anything fundamentally wrong with my personality or that I was basically neurotic. I was just in the process of reaction.

At approximately this time I heard from Nick that as part of her campaign of character assassination Enid had made a false accusation that I had been up to her room with a knife. I guessed that was a reference to the time I went up to her room in perfect innocence before scratching my wrists which led to her inviting me to tea. She had been talking to a German lecturer, an admirer of hers; he wrote her poetry and I surmised she had just wanted to impress the lecturer. He had been the one who told Nick. Nick told him that not everything Enid said was to be believed so I was not unduly worried by the lie.

But her attitude still led me to see her in a negative light and one day, when there was a front page headline in the paper, Devil Woman, about a woman who had got her two lovers to kill her husband, I cut it out, placed it in an envelope and put it in Enid's pigeonhole. The woman was wanton and her lovers followed her about like lapdogs. She reminded me of Enid who had turned my apparently near death from a so-called suicide attempt for which she was partly responsible, into a roaring joke. But though I saw her as evil I did not see her as anything more than down to earth. And this was my only contact though Nick retrieved the envelope.

One day I was walking past the window of Enid's room when I suddenly thought of her, not as human any longer, but subhuman because that was how she regarded me. It was a momentary thought and I did not express it to anyone but really I still thought of her as possessing the sanctity of a human being. I went up to John's room and expressed my disillusionment and frustrations to him. I had previously spoken to him a great deal about my self-image but he now refused to show understanding. He did however encourage me in a couple of hostile thoughts towards Enid. I no longer felt much anger though my talk was once or twice bitter. I recalled John's favourite joke at school, that of sawing off peoples arms and legs and was just very briefly (in four or five seconds) playing up to him, not because I had any remote idea of hurting her but because I wanted to see his reaction. That is everything and to say anymore would be an evil lie.

On a second visit to John's room he suddenly started to go off at a tangent with a sermon on the evils of homosexuality though he didn't define these. He thought that Ray should be locked up for life as should all homosexuals. I was amazed by how passionate and deep-rooted his aversion was to such people and was tempted to wonder if he thought of me as one. I looked back to our friendship at school and my mock hero worship of him. My natural physical distaste for the male physique meant I was never seriously able to think of myself as homosexual whatever any possible suggestion. John incapable of understanding me, may then have come to the false conclusion that I was as such (though that seems dubious) and I now had to consider if his hatred of Ray also indicated a hatred of me. Clearly John was not going to be of any help.

I determined to visit an ex-psychiatric nurse, the student who had been dancing with Ray at the beginning of the first term. He had asked me to come and discuss my sundry difficulties at any time. He was now notorious for his sexual behaviour in the university. His room was on the ground floor of Lloyd Thomas Hall where he used to "service" effeminate members of the homosexual clique and it stunk of excrement as did the neighbouring bathroom. I made myself comfortable in an armchair. The ex-psychiatric nurse, broad and manly, sat on his bed. I told him that I was experiencing the strange phenomenon of only finding myself deeply attracted to four or five women in the university and asked him if this was a symptom of anything. In fact I liked other women in the university too and they occasionally displayed an interest in me but I was still just in the grip of my neurosis about perfection. The ex-psychiatric nurse began to go on about homosexuality as if that could be the only explanation. I got up and left with a no clearer understanding of myself.

I wrote a letter to Dr. H.. I wanted to establish the possibility of getting my original face back and so of being my old self again. His letter in reply, which arrived at the end of May, was indignant and offered no further hopes on that score.

I had never seriously thought of actual violence but now I had an illusion that I had nothing to lose by violence. I was not able to study effectively for the summer exams which were already upon the university and I was wondering what there was left for me to do. My two suicidal gestures had only succeeded in arousing the contempt of people. I determined upon a more dramatic one. I thought of an expedition up to Enid's room with Tony's gun. A faith in me was nearly extinct but I retained a Christian set of morals. It was to be no more than a demonstration. However a gun would force the issue, the one thing people would heed.

Before I did anything I went back to Devon for a weekend. I rummaged round my bedroom in the vicarage for various photographs. Examination of the photographs would show the difference in me I thought. My parents drove me back to the university. After my parents had left I showed a few of the photos to my friends and gleaned their opinions. They agreed I had been done a disservice by my cosmetic surgeon. He had perhaps been over-confident with me instead of doing the bare necessary minimum. Nothing was now in the way of my plan. I have now written down every significant thought and action to this point including many that only I knew of.

CHAPTER 8
A FINAL CRY FOR HELP.

Just picking up the gun I knew would achieve nothing so I bought some cartridges in the ironmongers in Lampeter. These would give me that extra bargaining power I thought. It was the following Thursday that I put into effect the idea of trying to get hold of the gun from Tony's room and I dragged a builder's ladder a few hundred yards to prop up against his wall. I was spotted by someone on the balcony of Lloyd Thomas Hall so was obliged to run off and abandon the attempt. I thought about obtaining the gun again on the Friday but gave up the idea. On both occasions I was drunk. On both days I said to Tony: "I want to commit suicide" though I was not seriously thinking about it. On the Friday I also went up to John's room and dug into my jacket pocket for some cartridges which I showed him. I did not mention violence which wasn't on my mind. I guessed the cartridges might make him take me seriously. But for one more exam I could have walked out the university and all would have been well. No one did heed my plight.

The next Saturday Tony and I lay down on the lawn in front of Lloyd Thomas Hall in the sunlight. Before me resting on the grass were the Oresteia and the Iliad which I had to read through for Monday's exam, the one paper I needed to sit to pass my first year. I couldn't concentrate. I went off to the union bar and had three pints of cider. Then carrying a full pint glass of cider I walked out of the union bar to Tony's room. For the final time I said: "I want to commit suicide" though again that just reflected my mood, not intent. There was still no response. We remained together for a while saying nothing. After a few minutes had passed Tony said he had to go and see someone; I insisted on staying in his room while he was gone. He went off on his own.

In his absence I sought out the shotgun which I found concealed in a canvas guncase behind a bookcase. I grabbed the shotgun, took a back route out of Lloyd Thomas Hall through the rear carpark making for the stream and I hid the shotgun in some bulrushes. I emerged again and calmly walked back to Tony's room as if nothing had happened. I had done all that I had an inclination to do at that precise moment.

But as I had walked through the carpark, Richard, who had been looking through the window, had spotted me with the gun and went to raise the alarm. Tony returned to his room furious at having been told of the disappearance of the shotgun. I would have to run for it if I wanted to avoid a confrontation so made off.

As I was coming out of Lloyd Thomas Hall I bumped into Mark, Nick and a couple of other friends who had also been informed of the disappearance of the shotgun. Nick turned to the others and said:

"If Andrew wants to commit suicide let him."

They all lost interest in the subject of the lost shotgun, all that is except Tony and now Digby. As Tony still had to pay Digby for the gun, Digby was also angry over its disappearance. Indeed he stood to be disciplined for having it illegally on campus and he saw finding it as imperative. Seeing that at least Tony and Digby were after me and not of a frame of mind to do anything dramatic I just decided to get more drunk. I went into a supermarket in Lampeter and bought a bottle of Olde Englishe cider. Bottle in hand I returned to my room in the Terrapins where I consumed a quarter of it.

Tony appeared. He was still angry over the disappearance of the gun and I attempted to mollify him by saying that if he sold the gun to me he would be absolved of any responsibility should I kill myself, not that I thought things would come to that. He agreed to accept a cheque of £26 from me in payment for the gun. He appeared mollified.

After about a minute I walked out of the room and went for a pee in the toilet. But though Tony had appeared mollified I found him following after me and he even started to kick at the door of the toilet. I came out saying I was just going to get something from my room, disappeared inside and locked the door.

"Where is the gun?" Tony shouted from outside the room his anger rising.

"In a place you will never find it" I replied.

I was reluctant to tell him where I had hidden the shotgun for I still regarded it as the one lever left to me to influence peoples attitudes towards me. But though I still did not have any inclination to do anything dramatic I was being pressurised into acting. I thought of going up to Enid's room with the gun. First I resolved to set the campus ablaze. All in all I was planning to create a stir such as the university had never known before.

With a fleeting farfetched fantasy of getting myself shot by the police I went to my chest of drawers next to my bed and grabbed the remaining cartridges from the top drawer stuffing them into my jacket pocket. I accidentally left one of the twenty behind. There was no thought to hurt anybody.

My next concern was to escape Tony. I picked up my black shoulder bag off the floor, grabbed my bottle of cider, made for the window, opened it and climbed out dropping the shoulder bag inside as I jumped from the ledge outside to muffle the sound of my fall. I took to my heels, bottle in hand, taking an alleyway into the town and then following another route into the countryside. I edged my way round the back of the university campus and emerged behind the gymnasium near the half built building of John Richards Hall. I crept the hundred yards or so to the hall of residence and concealed myself in some bushes. A few minutes later I saw Digby and Tony striding angrily past the Arts building on the other side of the campus stream. I had only ruffled the feathers of two people, Digby and Tony.

I waited till they were out of sight and then left my hiding place and went into one of the uncompleted rooms in the hall of residence. I sat down on the floor in the corner, drew my cider bottle to my lips and started to swig at it. I mulled over my problems and how to overcome them but as usual came up with no answer. I started to cry but that did not help relieve my sadness. When I had finished crying and wiped the tears away I got up, left the building and walked a few yards ending up at John's hall of residence. I walked a little further and noticed an upstairs window in a hall of residence that had been broken. That gave me an idea. I went to Steve's window, a large sheet window on the ground floor, and knocked on it. Inside were Steve and his girlfriend. I said: "Do you want me to surprise you?" Steve said "yes" so I said: "Give me all the money in your money box then." His moneybox was on his desk and he emptied it into his hand. I pocketed the few pence it amounted to, removed the shoe from my foot and hit the window. With a second flick of the wrist I broke it carelessly dropping the shoe inside. I made off then bumped into John. I told him that I had broken two windows pointing at the one for which I was not responsible. He turned round and fled. I slowly made my way round Steve's and John's hall of residence and then entered the building climbing the stairs to John's room as I was curious to know where he had gone. I was still clutching my bottle of cider taking the occasional swig at it. John wasn't in his room and I took one of his slippers from his cupboard to put on my bare foot.

"I went into the boxroom to finish off my bottle of cider. As I swigged away I heard John calling downstairs:

"Has anyone seen Andrew Robinson?"

A little later I went back to John's room in the hope of finding him there so I could discuss the whole matter with him. I was not really of the frame of mind to go up to Enid's room with the gun even if my head was spinning from the effects of the alcohol. I had almost finished the cider though there was a drop left in the bottom of the bottle which I was still holding. In John's room I discovered not only him but Tony as well.

As I entered the room Tony reached out threateningly to grab me and as I was only two thirds his size I thought of the only weapon I had, the bottle, raising it above my head saying: "Tony, you are the last person in the world I want to hurt." I rather liked

112

him and certainly did not want to hurt him. I then backed to the door and hastened out of the room down the stairs.

Regrettably he and John decided to follow after me and were hot on my heels. I had shed the bottle. It was my last chance to act so I crossed the bridge over the stream and ran to the place where I had concealed the gun. By the time I reached the hiding place John and Tony were only thirty yards behind me. I grabbed the shotgun and popped in a cartridge from my pocket releasing the safety catch. I came out of the bulrushes roughly in the direction of Tony and John who were hesitating next to the Arts building. I took this route out because I had gone in that way and also because I hoped the sight of the shotgun would deter John and Tony from coming too close though I was careful not to point it at them. This was the limit of my thoughts and the sight of the shotgun in my hand did cause them to retreat.

I took aim at the base of a sapling growing nearby and fired to see how the gun worked for I was vaguely thinking of suicide though not seriously. (It was the show I was concerned with.) I had abandoned the idea of getting the police to shoot me as it was wildly farfetched and going up to Enid's room was all I really had in mind. I loaded the gun again and at that moment a professor shouted at me from his garden on the other side of the stream:

"What do you think you are doing you bloody idiot?"

I knew exactly what I was doing. I wanted to get people concerned and I was finally succeeding. The final stage in this process was to go up top Enid's room with the gun though there was no thought of physically harming her.

An acquaintance of mine was waving at me to go away from the bay window of the union building which lay en route to Enid's room and to discourage him from blocking my route I decided to trot rather than walk in the direction of the union building. All the time the shotgun remained pointed towards the ground. I felt no more dangerous than a car driver.

I soon covered the ground to the union building, clambered up the first flight of stairs on the way to the union offices, entered the quadrangle, hugged the inside of the main buildings as far as the entrance to Enid's sleeping accommodation area, passed Lorna's room on the ground floor where I noticed Lorna and Nick through the open door and mounted the stairs to Enid's room. I felt no malice and had no plans believing what I had done would create an effect.

Standing breathless on the landing outside her room I knocked on the door the shotgun lowered and the muzzle pointing at the floorboards. Enid opened the door and smiled. As usual she looked very pretty in the light of her room and it was her prettiness that I first noticed; her smile almost made me happy. The shotgun

113

remained lowered and pointing at the floor. There was no thought to raise it let alone pull the trigger.

Then she noticed the shotgun. Surprised she started back and said "no" and I stupidly gave the appropriate response "yes" though it was not said with seriousness and the shotgun remained lowered. But then she made to rush out at me on the landing and to try and prevent this I raised the barrel of the shotgun connecting her on the forehead with the muzzle. She ducked down beside me on my right and seized hold of the barrel of the gun with both hands. I had not expected this and just stood there unsure of what to do. Things were working out most unfortunately.

After four or five seconds I tried to move the gun but it remained useless, indeed a liability, in my hands. There was nothing I could have done to her even if had wanted to which I didn't. It was then that the expression on Enid's face changed to a mocking smile that clearly read: "Got you." It was a trap. I had been criminalised and I lost control trying momentarily to move the gun in her direction with my weak right hand moving right (two fingers was enough to counteract the momentary pressure on the barrel) knowing that hurting her was an impossibility and it was a simple matter for her to turn the gun away. I punched her on the head with my right fist; I was balancing the gun in my left hand. She cried: "Help me." The gun suddenly and accidentally discharged spraying the top of the bannisters on my left. A male and female student from the room next door hurried out and jumped on me, and I lashed out all about me. The gun had fallen to the floor and going on what was later written I might have made a half-hearted attempt to get hold of the gun again though such a thing would have been stupid as it was well nigh impossible and one of the girls threw the shotgun to the bottom of the stairs. Then I thought that if she had ruined my life I might as well hit her and so be punished for a little rather than nothing and I may have started tearing at her dress though I don't recall the photograph later showing any rips. Enid freed herself from the pile of bodies and ran downstairs followed by the other female student. I stopped turning and disentangled myself from the remaining combatant. I just stood there a little angry and thirty seconds later Nick, who had heard the rumpus, came up and said:

"You have gone too far this time."

I didn't know quite what he meant as up till this latest incident I had done nothing to Enid. I knew that if she had not reacted aggressively (She was never frightened, only angry), if she had cowered instead, if she had not smiled mockingly at that critical moment, there would not have been a struggle. And again if I had been able to hurt her I wouldn't have as it wouldn't have been a trap. I indicated this to Nick adding that things got "out of hand." Nick said referring to my nose: "It was not her fault." And I agreed.

114

But I expected it to be understood I only "lost my cool" when I discovered I was compromised and only when I knew there was no chance of inflicting serious injury on Enid. Nick and I walked into the room of the girl next door and I said to him:

"I've ruined my life."It was after all now a police matter and a few seconds later I said to him unnecessarily for the police had been called:

"You'd better call the police."

He said:"Come downstairs. I'll get Lorna to make you a cup of tea" as if a cup of tea would remedy the situation.

As he and I descended the stairs to Lorna's room I saw that he was a little shaky. In Lorna's room he asked Lorna to boil the kettle but she was slow in doing anything and seemed a bit shaky too.

I waited for my cup of tea but I saw it wasn't going to come so I climbed the stairs again followed by Nick and walked into Enid's room.

"Look what she's done to me now" I said of Enid frustration rather than anger welling up inside me and I moved to the desk, picked up the pot plants and books and threw them out of the window. I calmed down and waited placidly and resignedly by her desk for the police.

In three minutes the police arrived. In the confusion they thought Nick was the culprit as he had been walking round the room distractedly and they moved to arrest him. I had to say:

"It's me you want."

I was handcuffed and led down the stairs. Halfway down the staircase I said:

"I wanted to shoot Enid. I wanted to shoot Enid then kill myself."But these were just afterthoughts rather than any plans I had had. A policeman asked me why then I hadn't just picked up the gun at the bottom of the stairs and shot myself but in all my words I was just heated at having found myself criminalised. Enid was never in real danger and I was in fact just lost for words. If I had wanted to kill or maim Enid it would have been simple and those were not my thoughts or ideas.

We entered the quadrangle. The quadrangle was full of students. They had scurried out of their rooms like rabbits out of their burrows wondering what the disturbance was about. The main reason for this was that when the shotgun discharged it gave forth an exceptionally loud report. I covered my face with my free hand as if in shame though I wasn't sure if I felt any. Had I actually killed I know I would have felt terrible shame but I did not see what I had done as being very serious. Outside the quadrangle was a waiting police car and I was let in. The car drove off and I left the college forever.

At Lampeter police station I was locked in a cell. The cell was bare but modern and I was not unduly disturbed by my surroundings. But I had other worries and paced backwards and forwards with the thought of the terrible mess I had made of my life. I hadn't expected things to turn out remotely as badly but half an hour had made a tremendous difference to my life.

I noticed a little window in the cell which looked into the office and through it I observed what was happening. The police were in a great buzz of excitement and activity I had succeeded in creating a great stir and was now the subject of wild gestures and excited conversation. Obviously the Lampeter police had been bored for a long time and I had suddenly made their existences worthwhile and truly given them something to get their teeth into. But I had not meant to create quite such a stir.

Not liking what I was seeing I drew myself away from the window and started to pace back and forth, back and forth for what seemed an age. As there was no chair to sit on I could really do little else anyway.

After two hours I was brought a plate of sausages, chips and eggs and wolfed down the whole plateful. I had to confess I was surprised I should be provided with such an enjoyable meal and eating helped relieve the tension.

An hour later I was taken out of my cell, handcuffed and driven to Aberystwyth police station twenty miles away. It must have been about half past six that I was let out of my cell. On the journey I asked the policeman to whom I was handcuffed how long I would do inside.

"The previous bloke got four years." I didn't know that that case also involved Enid as I was later told rightly or wrongly.

The prospect of four years inside did not worry me and I remained calm. The policeman offered me a cigarette with the words:

"This is not allowed."

I took the cigarette, got a light off him and started to puff away. Despite his apparent show of kindness I realised he was listening intently to every word I had to say. I was careful not to say anything to incriminate myself.

A little later on the journey I said I would write a book on prison when I got out, but was told it had been done before and my attitude was seen as blase.

At Aberystwyth police station I was locked in a cell again but this time the cell had a toilet and a wooden bed. I sat down on the bed and contemplated my surroundings. I was not in luxury but the fact that there were people in the corridor meant that I did not feel totally alone and was thus stopped from brooding. I was however worried by how things had turned out and I again thought:

"What a bloody idiot I have been. "It was at this time that my parents were informed that I was in custody and they told the policeman who phoned them that they would be coming to see me as soon as possible. I later discovered they had been shattered by what they had been told.

Two hours later I was led up to the interrogation room. The two detectives who arrested me were going to interview me. They had no doubt been occupied with getting statements from people and were not in a pleasant mood. It was also apparent that they felt I had a bravado which needed to be knocked out of me, a bravado I didn't intend.

"Why did you want to kill this girl?" asked one detective.

I was not going to be verbalised and replied honestly: "I did not want to kill her." I in fact never ever admitted to such a thing.

"You have just had time to think about it. Why did you want to kill this girl?"

"I have told you I did not want to kill her."

"I have heard of guys knocking about their wives and girlfriends but they don't go out with a shotgun and try and kill them."

The other detective who was the soft man in the soft man hard man approach just sat back on the edge of a desk and watched the interrogation unfold. He hardly said a word for the first ten minutes.

"You gored Enid with the gun" said the aggressive detective.

"I did not" I replied.

"She received a semi-circular cut to her forehead."

I was puzzled; I didn't know I had physically hurt Enid. It was only later that I surmised that she must have received the semi-circular cut when I tried to prevent her from rushing out at me by raising the barrel of the shotgun.

The questioning continued with endless talk about killing by the aggressive detective and the occasional damaging remark from the other detective. Then, getting tired of the insinuations and also the serious accusations levelled against me I said to avoid needlessly and falsely incriminating myself:

"I will make a statement."

I had not been cautioned or informed of my rights and the quiet and placid detective and I sat down at a table facing each other. I was now very much at the mercy of the detectives. The quiet detective smoothed over a piece of paper and poised a pen above it. I thought for a minute or two then began to dictate. I was surprised that the recording of the statement was being done by the detective rather than me. The effect of this was that when we reached a point of controversy the pen would stop writing and only commence again when I agreed to say what the detectives wanted. For example when I said I had taken the shotgun from Tony's room the pen halted only resuming again when I substituted the word stole for the word took. As I was basically not a robber or a kleptomaniac and intended that Tony should have the gun back I only reluctantly yielded to the police on this point. I tried to press home my suicidal thinking but my depression was deemed irrelevant. When describing what happened on the landing outside Enid's room I was very confused and was guided into condemning myself totally unfairly with no chance to explain the trap (though I was too close to have seen it as such then) and that hurting her was an impossibility. Had I had any intention to hurt her the damage would have been done before. And I spoke a lot of rubbish to try and make a lesser charge of attempt to cause grievous bodily harm (which was also rubbish) to stick and so guard against a worse charge. My thoughts had not shaped themselves into a desire to kill and it had been purely a cry for help gone wrong though I was too close to the event to articulate such things. However bad my statement it did give an accurate chronology of events during the nine months I had been acquainted with Enid and after two and a half hours the dictating finally came to an end. The quiet detective ended by reading out my statement to me and after he had done so made me sign my name at the bottom. The two detectives yawned and stretched and called in another policeman to take me back to my cell. Only I felt wide awake.

After another half an hour in my cell a policeman appeared.

"Have you read my statement ?" I asked.

"Yes" he replied.

"What did you think of it?"

"It just seems like a very bad obsession to me." He was speaking of Enid.

As the policeman made to leave I asked him, as a complete afterthought if I could see a solicitor. He said he would telephone a Mr Griffiths.

Twenty minutes later Mr Griffiths arrived. He first went and read my statement and then he and I were given a little office in which to talk.

"You're not mad" he said perched on a chair behind the desk. Seated opposite him I said nothing. "Did you intend to kill this girl?"

"No" I replied.

I found his manner very warming and inspiring. He was middle-aged and obviously experienced in matters of violent crime. But at the moment he was clearly wanting to get back home and to bed for it was a late hour and after what was a short meeting he rose and left. I returned to my cell.

During the early hours of Sunday morning I snoozed a little and woke up to a fried breakfast of eggs, bacon, sausage, tomato and fried bread. I was hungry and would have happily wolfed down the lot, but I pretended not to have an appetite and so left my fine breakfast untouched. I had to feign guilt for although I didn't feel I had done anything to warrant guilt the police did not accept the truth of what had happened and I did not want to appear like a heartless monster to them by brazening it out. I had a deep conscience but that only stood to be fired when I did something seriously wrong. I had not killed anyone and I had not set out to do that.

That afternoon my parents arrived and a policeman let them into my cell. My mother sat down on the wooden bed beside me whilst my father remained standing.

"You're not a criminal" said my father "You're sick." He added: "It all goes back to the nose."

I thought that too but said nothing. I was not quite sure what to say to my parents. I had expected them to disown me. However,though my father was a man of the cloth and his reputation stood at risk, they had stuck by me even to this extremity.

After a while my parents left to go and find accommodation and then to go and see Mr Griffiths who had expressed a desire over the telephone to see them. They also wanted to see Mr Griffiths themselves to establish my prospects as far as the legal outcome of my case was concerned.

That afternoon my fingerprints were taken and the front and right profile of my face were photographed. I didn't mind this and treated it as routine. I was not even greatly disturbed to find myself locked up. "Stone walls do not a prison make" and my spirit roamed free. In fact at moments I felt quite exhilarated as a result of having exerted myself and the exhilaration hid the fear. That Enid sure in the prospect of happily married life had just been putting the finishing touches to her complete ruination of me was something I was unaware of so my exhilaration was not marred that way. And I did not fully realise then that I was now to be regarded by society as a criminal, that my chance in life had gone, that I was now scum.

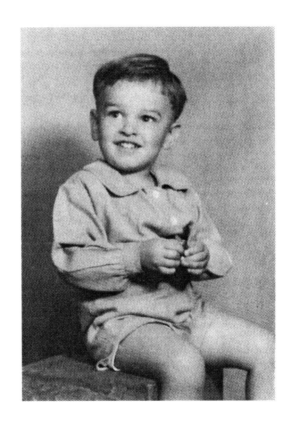

Aged 3-4

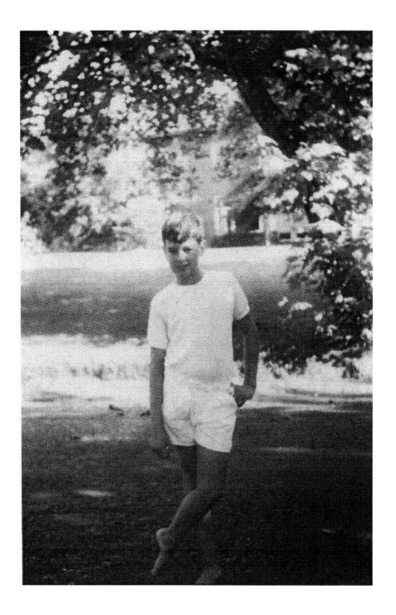

Aged almost 14

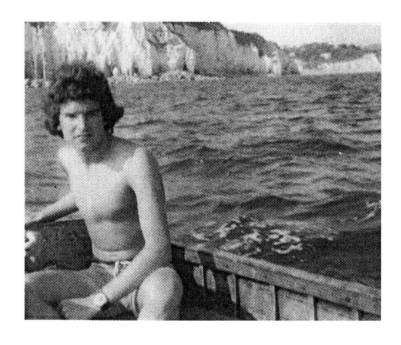

Before fully grown. Nose in perfect
proportion. Eyes screwed up by sun.

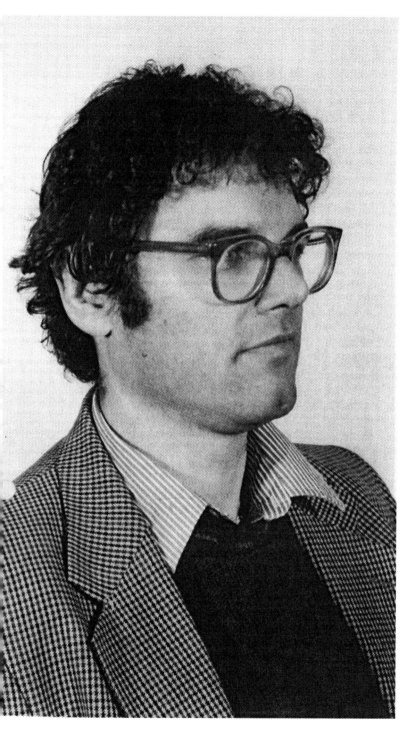

Now nose sticks out too much as clear to anyone with an aesthetic sense.

CHAPTER 9
THE PSYCHIATRIC OPTION.

I met Mr Griffiths on the Monday, June 5th 1978, at the magistrates court in Abaraeron and his manner was as warm and encouraging as ever. But I was bemused when I discovered that he wanted to send me to a hospital as the first thing he had said to me was that I was not mad. However he behaved as if what he was doing was routine and I could only assume that the idea was for me to prove myself sane but that I had been driven by abnormal pressures. That I should be diagnosed as mad or that I would end up in a hospital for a protracted period of time had seemed out of the question though that is not to say I did not want some help or guidance, the main reason for my going up to Enid's room with the gun.

So Mr Griffiths said to the magistrates that I had attempted suicide twice to reinforce the picture of me as a tragic figure which the nature of the charges suggested and despite police opposition I was bailed for one month to St. David's Hospital Carmarthen. The police were not happy about this for they thought that I might get off lightly but Mr Griffiths was all smiles. It was also decided that my parents, who were present in court, should drive me there.

After the hearing I left the court with my parents and we headed for Carmarthen through luscious green countryside. After an hour we reached the entrance to the hospital. Driving through the grounds I saw several "zombies" in overalls and with shaven heads raking the lawns. At the front entrance to the main buildings my parents got out of the car, went inside and enquired as to whether I was expected. Apparently I was not so they were advised to take me to the general hospital where I had been before. I was duly taken there and indeed I was expected there; my parents left and I was admitted into the psychiatric unit.

My parents had left a holdall full of clothes and other personal effects and carrying it I was shown to my bed by a female nurse and told to get into my pyjamas. A couple of female nurses appeared. I found myself the object of intense interest. I wasn't probed with questions; I was just stared at and in a way that suggested I was not a failure but a hero. I had been mentioned on the radio and in the newspaper and they knew about me.

Five minutes later the young doctor with the beard whom I recognised from my stay before, came to examine me. The curtains round my bed were drawn and I was asked to take off my pyjama top and lie down. I was prodded and probed and my heart beat was listened to. After the physical examination was over the doctor asked:
"Do you hear voices?"
"No" I replied truthfully.

"Do you think that people are plotting against you?"

"No" I said for I thought I had no reason to think that.

"Did this girl (Enid) ask you to marry her?"

Even now I was too bashful to answer the question.

"Did she taunt you over sex?"

The last question was significant but I was a little worried by some of the other questions. I was anxious enough to put a halt to the questioning for I did not want to be browbeaten or influenced in any way as to what I said. Words had to be used carefully and with so much at stake I did not want to mislead anyone by off the cuff replies so I said:

"I'll write down on paper for you a list of all the pressures I was under when I did what I did."

The young doctor left.

That same morning, after the nurses had vacated my bedside, I proceeded to do just that. To write the significant points down on paper seemed the most sensible thing to do and I amassed some twenty points down on paper including retrogressive nose operations, broken love affairs, loss of respect and credibility, slanders. I also mentioned pressure of work but omitted to say how I had been affected by all these things simply saying that I had "crying spells". My only conclusion was that my future appeared a blank. After completing the list I handed it in.

That afternoon I was allowed back into my day clothes and moped about the ward for the rest of the day. I discovered a snooker table downstairs, picked up a cue and potted a few balls. I still felt isolated and my life was devoid of excitement. But I made the most of my time on the ward and did speak to one female nurse who had a pretty face though she was plumpish. She did take some interest in me but when my mind wasn't on my legal position it was on Enid. My legal position had the effect of a nagging doubt rather than a deep worry and my performance was not impaired by that side of things.

The next day I appeared in front of the three doctors, the young doctor, Dr. E. and the older and wiser doctor, all whom I remembered from my previous stay on the ward. My consultant, Dr. E. said:

"We thought you would be more comfortable here than at St. Davids."

That at least made me think the doctors must have my best interests at heart.

"Why did you do it?" Dr. E. asked.

I assumed he was referring to why I went up to Enid's room with the gun.

"I have given you a list of twenty things that influenced me to do what I did" I said. "I'll go through each point in turn if you

121

like." I also assumed the doctors and my solicitor would be exchanging information so did not bother to duplicate it, a terrible mistake as it turned out.

"Dr. E. replied: "We know what you have written but why did you do it?"

I was dumbstruck. After that I wondered what more I could say. I had written down the main factors and I had written the truth. Beyond that I thought that all that was left open to me was to use my imagination. But the idea of concocting a defence based on lies did not occur to me. I believed everybody else bar Enid would be telling the truth as well.

"We are looking for malice" said the young doctor.

Establishing truth and justice had seemed so simple a matter and suddenly the young doctor had spoken of malice and so complicated the whole issue. At some stage there had been slight malice, understandable malice I thought. But I wondered why it was being treated as the most important issue. My defence which was perfect had been removed right from the start and I was never able to repeat it. Psychiatrists worked in a mysterious way. When I walked out of the office it was with certain doubts.

The next day I was blessed with a visit from my tutor. He was a very sympathetic person who had both understanding and insight. He was a senior French lecturer and used to invite me along to the occasional party with others majoring in French where in the first term Lorna used to ask me to dance. Of course he had been apprised of my two "suicide attempts" and thought of me as a congenial individual who suffered from bouts of depression. He did not see me as violent and saw the shotgun incident as a bid to attract attention which it was or a suicidal gesture. Even now I was having suicidal thoughts though I was not in danger of killing myself and I discussed them with him though he urged me against suicide adding that suicide can cast a pall over many peoples lives. It was essentially a moral issue though I could only think of two people whom my possible suicide would hurt, my mother and my father. But I was grateful to my tutor for his concern.

The next day my mother came down from Devon to visit me. As she had come such a long way the sister gave her permission to visit me whenever she liked and for as long as she liked instead of just ordinary visiting hours. I had been placed all on my own in one part of the ward and there my mother and I sat. At that stage my feelings of sadness had begun to affect me deeply and I strongly sensed my isolation. My mother put her arm round me for comfort when I started to weep. Only my mother witnessed my tears. Most of the time I was fairly bright; the nurses who had seen me on the ward the previous November remarked on how improved I seemed.

Only my mother knew the truth, that I had reached another trough and the doctors were not even properly aware of my depression.

When I was on my own I began to wallow in my depression. Then, as I was lying on my bed one afternoon, I experienced a strong momentary anger towards Enid. I thought of her sitting her exams and had a desire to seize a knife and do her harm. It was the rebound affect to what I was feeling but was the only time I felt such a thing and was the final acknowledgement that I had been ruined romantically and academically. At this time I did not even regard such feelings as relevant. It was not that I wanted to hide the truth. It was just that over a period of nine months under intense pressure and provocation I had felt very little anger indeed.

I had one more visit and a letter from my tutor but then Enid slandered me to him and that was the last I heard from him. I also had a visit from the chaplain of St. David's University College and the newly elected president of the students union there, a female. But I had a mild sense of shame along with a fear of being misunderstood and therefore did not know if I wanted visitors.

Then a visit occurred, a visit I didn't expect, but one of more import. It was from Julie and Ray.

"You look amazingly calm" Julie said slumped on a bed opposite me.

"Why shouldn't I be?"

"Well everyone has made statements to the police and they seem bent on getting you the worst sentence possible."

"Oh, come on" I exclaimed. "What's there to say?" And though I recalled the things I had said to people on that my sentiments were totally genuine.

"Enid got everyone together in her room to decide what they should say before making their statements" said Julie. "Then they trooped off to the police station laughing. It was like a James Bond movie."

Despite the faults of my "friends" I didn't believe they would go out of their way to destroy me so I said:

"My friends are an honest enough lot aren't they?"

"John walked out of the police station saying he hoped to see you locked up in four thick walls for the rest of your days."

Digby as well as John had been expelled from schools; Digby had smashed up a telephone booth, but I still did not believe John would go out to do me harm. I knew he preyed on weakness and that he used to mock the afflicted at school but I believed that was just schoolboy jesting and did not think he would wantonly ruin my life. I remembered his recipe for Ray and his like: "They should be locked up for life" but I still trusted in his overall integrity. I was completely unperturbed by Julie's words. Ray said he spoke to Enid after the incident saying that if I had wanted to shoot her why didn't

I do it when she opened the door? I had had ample opportunity then had that been my intention which it was not. After Julie and Ray had left I concluded Julie had just got things out of proportion.

A little later Julie sent me a love letter. She obviously admired me and thought that going up to Enid's room with a shotgun was not only a brave thing, she said I was brave to have done it, but the only thing I could have done in the circumstances. It was nice to have her support.

At this time a blonde girl with beautiful features was admitted onto the ward. In the lounge she offered me a cigarette. I declined and though she too was very friendly to me I did not respond as I did not want the responsibility of associating with a beautiful girl. She had taken an overdose and was due to go to Germany. After she had left I heard she had taken another overdose.

At the end of my second week at "Carmarthen General Hospital" a girl appeared on the ward who was going to make me revise my whole outlook. She was tall, well covered, erect with long brown hair, a regular jaw, a straight nose and deeply set eyes. She was not beautiful but she had a strength and self-assurance that greatly attracted me just then. I found myself gazing at her which was significant as up till now I had only deeply fancied women with traditionally beautiful facial features. Despite a steady flow of patients through the ward this new patient was the only one I considered. Carrying the girls bags was a man of about fifty five and a blonde-haired good looking man of about twenty two.

In the afternoon as I was sitting alone in the lounge the girl entered and sat down in the chair opposite me. The lounge was small with old shabby vinyl armchairs, some with gashes, lined across opposing walls. But I was oblivious to my surroundings finding myself only interested in the girl opposite.

"Do you want to commit suicide with me?" she asked.

I was taken aback by the question, but I felt an instant rapport with her. She had an intuitive understanding of me and a deep sympathy for my outlook which only a fellow sufferer could feel. I asked her why she wanted to commit suicide. I was more amused than puzzled. She explained that her marriage was in pieces and that she didn't love her husband. I suggested she find someone else but though she had tried other men she was not able to feel for them either. I said that I too couldn't love anyone who loved me but that I did love someone who didn't love me. We talked about love and our joint problem which in the end boiled down to, not being incapable of finding someone, but of finding someone we could love. I even wondered whether the girl was making some kind of invitation.

That evening, when the other patients had gone to bed, I found myself sitting in the lounge opposite the girl. She said her name was Barbara and she said the middle-aged man carrying her bags was her father, the blonde-haired young man, her brother. She had a slightly ruddy complexion and her voice was husky but her manner made me warm towards her. Barbara then moved from her chair sitting down next to me. We sat there for a few minutes saying very little. She was resting her arms on the arms of her chair; my right arm was resting next to hers on the arm of my chair. I moved my hand so that it rested on top of hers and as I did so I experienced a warmth pass from her hand up my arm to my heart. For the first time in three months I felt the pain in my breast ease and my depression go. There was a chemistry between us, a meeting of two minds. I had not discovered the fleeting paradise I found with Enid but I had discovered something on which to build.

The next day Barbara and I spent much time together. We had a lot to say to one another and went for a walk round the hospital grounds. The sun shone brightly and the sky was a perennial blue. The leaves on the trees were a fresh green, not yet despoiled by the summer sun and the birds in the trees continued their singing. I was at last happy.

But the doctors were not so happy for though I had seen them almost everyday they were still no nearer explaining the charges. And all the time they kept on saying they were looking for malice. Fearing I would be seen as a cold-blooded monster if I said nothing I said in the end that I felt a "slow anger" though at that stage it had all gone. They then asked me where this anger came from but as they had rejected my initial reasons I was lost for an answer. When asked my intentions I stupidly said I had an idea of "scarring" Enid as I did not think I would be believed if I said I was just out for attention, the truth. My suicidal ideas and my desire to find a way out were not mentioned.

A day or two later Barbara said to me as we were walking down the main corridor of the ward:

"I don't care what you've done Andrew."

"Have you been talking to the doctors?" I asked.

"Yes."

"And what did they say?"

"Only that you've got problems and that I should stay well clear of you."

"And what did you say?"

"I said you were the only person I felt happy with."

I was pleased that the misunderstandings and interference of the doctors should not have disturbed such harmony and they had not succeeded yet in destroying what existed between us. But I was beginning to get worried by the wrong conclusions they were obviously starting to draw about me. I was beginning to doubt that they had any real concern for my well-being and assumed they had just been pressurised into accepting me by my solicitor. I did say "a terrible miscarriage of justice is being done."

During that week the blonde-haired young man with Barbara when she first went into hospital turned upon the ward with two very attractive children. The sight of the children caused me to think a little. Only then did I realise the man wasn't her brother after all but her husband. It did not look good for me to be associating with a married woman before my trial and Barbara's husband could not have been too happy either. But I was happy in her company and had no intention of discarding her which would have helped no one. Though she was married she was an important ally and I needed all the allies I could get.

Mr Griffiths came to see me on the ward. He sat down in front of a desk in an interview room.

"If you knew what you'd said in your statement to the police you'd be shocked" he chirped. His manner was deceptively warm and reassuring. I knew exactly what I'd said in my statement though I did not say this to him. Then he said as if this was my only defence:

"You cracked."

The comment surprised me as I had never considered that I had cracked before though the enormous pressures I was under were no doubt behind my action which wasn't reflective of my normal self. Mr Griffiths who never liked to clutter his clients minds with words advised me in a fairly vague manner not to go to open court but to have everything settled out of court. With those words he rose and left. He was the very incarnation of hope. But his advice was too brief and inexact and he was more of a reassuring presence than a counsellor. But my confidence remained intact though it seemed to avoid a legal fiasco I would have to literally take his advice.

Once he had left I thought deeply about his comments. I had "cracked" so I had been told. Putting that another way it seemed I had to admit to an uncontrollable feeling of malice and in turn plead lack of responsibility for my action. I decided that in a small way I would try and fit in with the doctors and I went back to my bed, took a pad of letter writing paper out of my locker and wrote the nonsense statement that "the volcano had to erupt"and that I had felt a compulsion "to go up to Enid's room with a loaded gun." I placed the sheet of paper in an envelope and left it in the doctors interview room for the doctors to read.

With my situation becoming dire the nurses began to offer alternative advice. Principally they suggested I should say I remembered nothing about what had happened on the day of my arrest but I felt the advice dangerous.

Near the end of my third week on the ward Julie entered the picture again. She it emerged, was a psychiatric patient herself. Obviously both she and Ray knew what it was like to be an outsider and could thus sympathise with me. She had apparently bumped into Dr. E. and had mentioned to him that I had been ragged in public in a rather horrible way about my new appearance. In fact all it had amounted to was a little gentle teasing which was confined to a few friends. But seeing that no progress had been made with me she had even written to Mr Griffiths. In her letter to him she had not only described the so-called teasing in public but had gone onto describe the fantasies of those who wanted to get me convicted of attempted murder and gave this as the reason. In fact the only thing they had to go on was my perfectly justifiable anger at having had my so-called suicide attempts turned into a joke, something I had as said discovered a month into the summer term at Lampeter. And Julie had spoilt all her good work by writing the lies and inaccuracies of the prosecution case. I never read the letter till much later.

If Julie's letter was thus unacceptable as evidence for the defence, the doctors believed that in Julie's words they could now explain the charges. So they pressed me to say I had been turned into an "object of public derision". Dr. E. said that had he been teased in public in the same way he would have been very angry. But I still had not been angered by the teasing seeing teasing as a common enough phenomenon amongst people especially children and did not want to put the blame onto my friends. I even thought it would have been unethical to do so. I read something much later which I certainly didn't say that I had been humiliated in public because of Enid for a year and she had become a symbol to me which I had wanted to attack, though it was total nonsense that such a thing was actually true and that I had been angered by it. The idea I discovered was not to help but destroy me.

Then Tony visited me and we stood chatting in the lobby downstairs. I said that I was in control when I went up to Enid's room with the gun and his thoughts were: "Were you?" I added that the doctors wanted me to blame it on my friends ragging me in public over my appearance and he replied:"We can say that if you want." It did seem that his crowd was not badly disposed towards me.

After that I became the subject of a case conference attended by a nurse, a few psychologists and several psychiatrists. It was held in the lounge downstairs. When I was called in I was again simply asked: "Why did you do it?" There was evidently now no doubt in the eyes of everyone present that I was guilty over the charges that I faced though it was much later I realised psychiatrists only worked for the prosecution and were not remotely interested in truth or justice. Dr. E. did try and help by suggesting that I had been made angry by the result of the nose refinement though of course I had been made depressed rather than angry on that score. I did hear on the television that the effect of making a man's nose smaller was psychological emasculation and thus depression was the logical result. I would have liked to have spoken about my former depression but nobody was prepared to listen. The case conference achieved nothing.

The next day I was hauled into the interview room by the young doctor who asked me with a note of urgency in his voice if I had been turned into an object of public derision. "It's your head on the chopping block" he warned me. I was still determined not to sacrifice my principles for the sake of an acquittal or light sentence.

After my refusal to take this way out I became hated by all and sundry. I was told by the doctors that they did not want me back after my pending court hearing and that I had only been accepted for the purpose of assessment, not treatment. My interviews with the doctors were rounded off with a few irrelevant questions, one of which was how I regarded men. I had talked about my worship of physical beauty and in consequence that if a good-looking man walked into the room I would look up. I did not say I was homosexual which I was not. I was just obsessive about physical beauty though I did not say I had discovered a favourable response to a woman not in the traditional mould beautiful. And the doctors in no way appreciated my improvement. The discussion amongst the doctors began to revolve more about my sexual identity than my perfectionism.

I was told by the young doctor that the report had been written and that the doctor's conclusion was final. I knew that I would be going to prison. I could have avoided prison had I decided to compromise on my principles but I had dangerously stuck to the truth in which I believed. But I thought my friends would be telling the truth in their statements too and that both sides of the story would emerge. I was not frightened of four years inside but thought that with the testimony of my friends it would be much less.

I told Barbara that I was going to prison. She became concerned over the fact that I was associating with her because she was married and wondered if that was the reason why the doctors had, like Pontius Pilate, washed their hands of me. The young doctor said that that was not the case.

I phoned Mr Griffiths from the callbox downstairs. He had received a copy of the report but did not tell me what had been written in it. He just said that it gave him nothing to "hang up" his "hat on." He had wanted me to be freed on section 1 which would have meant showing a satisfactory psychiatric report to a judge in chambers. I had put a spanner in the works by not implicating my friends. I didn't know that it was the opinion of doctors that if you committed a crime there had to be something wrong with you psychologically. Although men often raped, pillaged and killed in war because you were given a licence to do so, in peace time you could do nothing without a label being pinned onto you though in effect I had been involved in a war. And I was given my label, personality disorder. It was better to be considered a personality disorder than mad. But the doctors had decided to destroy me by writing at the end of the report that they couldn't guarantee that I wouldn't do the same thing again. Rubbish. They had also gone out of their way to get me convicted of the worst charges I faced ignoring my own statements and using any falsehood they could. Though they mentioned my "suicide attempts" they hardly mentioned my former depression speaking only of a mythical anger, adding that I was incurable, all nonsense. The only good thing they said was that I was "highly intelligent".

During my third last evening on that ward I waited for the police to come with the court summons. I waited in vain because Mr Griffiths had told them not to bother me. It had become his policy to shield me from the truth. I was not even told the "police statements" were due out though I expected them any day.

The next night the police statements came out. Mr Griffiths comment on the phone was that they did not " paint a pretty picture". My parents had not read them but they had obtained a copy of the psychiatric report and my father had shown it to a Dr. Pears in Exeter. She had said she could "cure" me. Mr Griffiths had different plans.

That same evening my parents drove up from Devon and collected a copy of the police statements from Mr Griffiths before visiting me. I sat down in the waiting room and began to read them. I was shocked to discover in the first line of John's statement that he was trying to make out I wanted to get a gun, not because of vague suicidal notions, the truth, but because I wanted to kill Enid, a total lie. He alleged that I thought Enid was literally a witch, absolute nonsense and that before going up to the landing outside her room with the gun I had stormed into his room brandishing my cider bottle above my head like a madman adding that I was totally paranoid. All that was rubbish; I had been drunk but calm and had only raised the bottle when Tony, who was in the room and much bigger than me, had threatened me and Tony fortunately quoted me then in his statement: "You are the last person the world I want to hurt." John also said that my meeting with Enid in the spring term was arranged in the spring term with Enid because I was hostile to her, a falsehood. It was arranged because I had cut my wrists through reactive depression. Digby, annoyed that I had taken his shotgun from Tony's room had collaborated with John agreeing with him on that also implying that when I looked at his shotgun at the beginning of the summer term I smiled because of a sinister motive. In fact I had forgotten about Enid at that stage and was just relieved in having found a way of ending my depression. Turning back to John's statement, I took in an additional lie, namely that I had shot at him and Tony. Whatever support Tony might have tried to give on this, the truth was I had not fired the gun at them, only at the base of a sapling which fortunately the police photographed. Enid made me out to be a mad dog saying that when I went up to her room with the gun my eyes were "white" and that but for her" quick reaction" I would have killed her, absolute nonsense. Tony in his statement also mentioned the occasion we spread a pamphlet out about guns on his desk but he did not mention my desire for a way out in suicide, the truth. And at that time I had forgotten about Enid. Nick was just out to cover for Lorna and though he knew the full story of what had happened said nothing. Most of the remaining statements said what Enid told the other witnesses to say, namely that I had been continuously angry instead of depressed and that I was threatening instead of self-destructive, the truth. For example both Enid and the girl in the room next door to her said that I had stood outside her room for fifteen minutes on the evening I cut my wrists. As seen I had only stood there for two minutes. To get the length of time to tally and so make the visit seem sinister which it wasn't the girls had agreed upon the time of fifteen minutes. Clearly everything had been twisted around. It was a witchhunt. I rose, turned to my parents heartbroken then with the full knowledge that God was dead and that for me the world had come to an end, I walked out of the waiting room into the charge nurse's office. I said: "I don't believe it" and collapsed in a dead faint on the floor still holding the statements.

The following night, my last night at "Carmarthen General Hospital", Barbara and I decided upon a celebration. It was my last night of freedom and I just wanted one more taste of living before I went to prison. The circumstances were just right because I had got over my depression and I was not frightened of prison despite Julie's warning that I would be made someone's woman. And we decided to go to the pub down the road. As we walked Barbara suggested we run away, but even if I was breaking the conditions of my bail by leaving the hospital grounds, I was not of the opinion we should do anything as drastic as that. I just wanted to enjoy myself while I had the chance and I did not think that running away would solve anything. I had already braced myself to fight the pack single handed in court. My only worry was that dirt tactics appeared to be the order of the day.

At the pub I ordered a pint of cider, Barbara a pint of beer. We moved to a quiet corner and started to sip our pints. I watched her swallowing hers which she did like an experienced drinker. I was pleased that she too liked to live it up. She was talkative saying how much she preferred me to her husband and a sailor boyfriend. After our first pint we refilled and moved to a more crowded part of the pub. On the bench next to us was a man of about forty drinking a pint of beer and Barbara said something ridiculous to him about us being trapeze artists from a nearby circus or something. Actually quite funny. She possessed an aggressiveness in her approach to people which I lacked although I did not read anything into this at the time. I was just happy to have met someone who was prepared to defy the world, even stand up for me. It was almost as if she was trying to impress me. Then the whole evening was shattered by a voice over the tannoy:

"Will Andrew Robinson please report to the back door."

We rose, left our pints and went to the back door where we discovered two policemen. Outside was a police van. For some reason I could never get away with anything. But this time I had a defence in the shape of Barbara and she said to the policemen:

"It was all my fault, honest. I begged him to come out with me."

"Get into the back" ordered one of the policemen and Barbara and I climbed into the back of the police van. Back at "Carmarthen General Hospital" we had to sit in the waiting room while the nurses considered what to do. After about ten minutes we were called into the charge nurse's office.

"Your husband has been worried sick about you" a nurse said to Barbara. "You have no right to walk out of the hospital just as you please."

Barbara said nothing.

"Now what have you got to say for yourself Andrew?" said a second nurse.

"Nothing" I said.

"It was all my fault" Barbara added.

"Both of you have been behaving like two little children" said a third nurse.

"It wasn't Andrew's fault" repeated Barbara.

I wanted to burst out laughing. My life had become a tragi-comedy and at that moment I couldn't fail to see the funny side. My face broadened into a smile but Barbara gave me such a damning look I thought better of it and assumed a serious countenance.

"We had to phone the police" the sister said and she explained the conditions of my bail which I already knew but which I couldn't take seriously now that authority appeared like a little child wielding power.

The nurses ordered Barbara and me to bed as if we were two little children and with much fuss and bother she went off in one direction and I, meek as a lamb, in the other.

The next morning I woke up to the thought that that day I would be going to prison. I also knew I would be saying goodbye to Barbara. I had no intention of subjecting her to the ignominy I now had to face by asking her to stick by me.

At breakfast I sat at the same table as Barbara but did not mention prison. After breakfast I penned a quick note to her saying I was not her ideal man in bed (though I might have been) and that I was not as handsome as I used to be. Also that Enid, whom I hadn't mentioned before, was evil. I didn't want her to be surprised should she read about my case in the newspaper. I gathered the remainder of my things and took them to the top of the stairs on the ward. There I waited with Barbara for my parents. Only when they arrived did I hand the note over to Barbara telling her not to read it until I had left. I picked up my holdall and carried it to my parents car.

We left Carmarthen General Hospital at about ten o'clock and drove to Abaraeron with few pressing doubts and in a calm atmosphere. Our entire approach was fatalistic but my father was apprehensive about my being thrown into a world of homosexuals and murderers. I myself was not too worried about that even though the word murderer still sent a cold shiver down my spine. Despite the fact that some of my so-called friends and enemies had made me out to be as bad as a murderer I could in no way think of myself like that. As I could not conceive of myself as capable of murder I had almost begun to believe that other people would in the end see me for what I was, harmless.

CHAPTER 10
THE CHAMBER OF HORRORS.

At Abaraeron Magistrates Court I was met by three policemen in the entrance. I noticed the chaplain of St. David's University College, the president of the students union, a middle-aged woman reporter in the gallery and my solicitor and the prosecution solicitor in the well of the court. Before the proceedings I started to chat with the policemen. Despite the mountain of fabricated evidence against me I had not been cowed and I even dug into my holdall producing the slipper I had borrowed from John's room handing it to the policemen with the words: "One stolen slipper." Again I was saying with irony that I did not take things that did not belong to me for personal enrichment like the thief.

On entering the interior of the court I moved over to my solicitor. In my hand I had a few notes and Mr Griffiths seized them with much earnestness as if they might hold the key to my freedom. Even as I handed them over I knew that there was nothing in them that would change anything though they revealed my former depression. Mr Griffiths then had a word with the prosecution solicitor saying of my statement to the police: "For goodness sake, this statement was written for him." He was obviously worried to still be questioning my statement but though it contained a lot of damning rubbish, notably towards the end, it did something to forestall the accusations of the pack and I did not know that he had just told my parents that things had become "very serious indeed". I myself commented to the policeman next to me that I thought the statements were very unfair and biased. He replied that he was "satisfied" they had been given in "good faith ", but he would. It was the first time I realised that lies were a fully accepted tool in a court of law.

During the hearing Mr Griffiths said to the magistrates that I had been on sleeping tablets for I had been on them at "Carmarthen General Hospital"; the idea was that I see another psychiatrist who could write another report favourable to me for the present one was liable to be the final thing to destroy me.

At the end of the hearing I was remanded in custody for one week in Cardiff Jail. The police and the pack had had their way. But the chaplain and union president both gave encouraging smiles and I was still so trusting that I thought the police, who after all belonged to the best police force in the world, would treat me fairly in the end. Just before I left the court building Mr Griffiths said in a voice both urgent and insistent: "You must stop protecting your friends. Just think what bastards they have been." Obviously he wanted me to turn the tables and blame everything on my friends teasing me in public over my nose. I just contemplated trying to disprove every accusation against me in court. I was then handcuffed to a policeman and led out of the court building, a policeman following behind with my holdall.

I was squashed into the back of a police car between two policemen. Two sat in front. The car drove off, we passed through green countryside and I looked ahead to the unknown. Until a week ago I had simply expected a short rigorous spell in prison, the disgrace of being brought before the public eye, the ruination of my university career. Now there was the real fear I might be in all the newspapers and end up with a life sentence. But I remained calm and I was still determined to fight my case according to the rules laid down by the law, not according to the gutter, like my enemies.

After an hour's drive we arrived at Cardiff Jail and its gates were opened by some prison officers impressively dressed in blue uniforms and caps. Inside directions were given to the reception area and we drove the few yards there. I took in my new home. The prison was surrounded by a high wall with barbed wire running along the top broken by watch towers. The main buildings of the prison were of grey stone and consisted of row upon row of little barred windows.

At the reception area I was handed over to the prison authorities and made to change into prison dress. An inventory was made of all my belongings by a prison officer and I had to hand in my watch and all personal effects for storage. Afterwards I sat down on a bench amidst several detainees, all young. A convict came over and gave me a quick vocabulary and arithmetic test to do. I found my mind wandering so that I wrongly answered the most simple questions and when he returned a couple of minutes later he took great delight in pointing out one ridiculous error.

A convict with a "cocky" air instructed me to have a bath. I stripped and stepped in and was just grateful that the water was hot. No sooner had I begun to relax and enjoy it than a rasping voice cut through my tranquillity: "Hurry up you scum." It suggested firstly that I was the enemy and secondly that though not yet tried I was guilty. Contrary to what I had once believed you were guilty until proven innocent. Seeing that my punishment had already started and fearing a worse one if I didn't respond immediately I jumped out of the bath and without bothering to dry myself dragged on my clothes. I joined the batch of about ten prisoners presided over by a man in a suit with piercing eyes whom I understood to be the doctor, a doctor with a Sergeant Major like command of the situation. We set off down a dimly-lit passageway after the doctor.

We came to a halt outside the surgery. We were made to line up in a queue, the doctor entered the surgery and the first in the queue was ordered in. As I was waiting the prisoner just ahead of me turned to me and said: "I'm in here for driving offenses. I'm taking the can for three others. But I don't mind. In fact I like prison." Had I expected a minor sentence I too may have found prison an exciting adventure. It was impossible now to think of it as enjoyable or funny.

Quickly the queue dwindled and my turn came to enter. Inside I had to strip and the doctor gave me a cursory examination, its perfunctory nature explaining why the other prisoners had been dealt with so quickly. Afterwards a kindly-faced prison officer took me aside and asked if a psychiatric report had been made on me. On replying in the affirmative he said: "Then there will be no more psychiatric reports." I replied "yes" though deep down I had a sickening feeling of doubt as I thought my only chance of a fair trial lay in a satisfactory psychiatric report. I was asked if I had attempted suicide and I said "yes". When asked how I stupidly replied: "I put the muzzle of a shotgun to my head and placed my toe on the trigger." It was not true but as I was not slandering anyone by saying such a thing I saw no harm in it and faintly hoped it might lead to a referral to the hospital wing where I though I might find both comfort and justice. In reality I would have been well advised to deny any suicidal thoughts. Another prison officer was summoned by telephone from the hospital wing and in no time at all he appeared. He was short and fat with a Machiavellian face and evil black eyes. He gave me a sinister smile before ordering me to follow him.

We set off through another door passing through another dimly-lit passage. We entered a room where some young convicts were watching television. We moved on passing through another door and in addition to the sound of locking and unlocking the prison officer made a continual show of jangling his keys as if to remind me of my lost freedom.

We entered a passage on either side of which were thick studded doors painted a glaring orange. Slotted in the doors at head height were grills as of a medieval dungeon and behind the grills, pressed to the bars, I saw faces, faces drained of any hope. To make it worse was the feeling that mingled with this all-pervasive misery was the powerful presence of evil, of caged up evil wanting to break out, of evil that spread like a foul exhalation through the whole passage. It was all like something out of a horror movie. Somehow I succeeded in shutting out the truth of what I was witnessing and hoped that in no time I would be out of the passage and in what I envisaged the hospital wing would be, a place of warmth and comfort. But at a cell door three quarters of the way down the passage my escort suddenly stopped.

"Here we are " he smiled opening the cell door.

I realised with a sudden dread that this passage was the hospital wing.

As I entered the cell I observed that it was completely bare but for a foam mattress, two blankets and a chamber pot in the corner. The cell door then clicked shut behind me and I saw my whole world diminish into nothing, into this bare cell. I looked about my cell, about my future home, and saw how cramped it was. It was eight feet by twelve. The only window was a tiny aperture covered with glass high upon the wall opposite the door affording a scanty view of grey sky. Above was a white light which could be turned to orange by pressing a switch next to the door. There was also an alarm button. The walls were otherwise bare and white as if to emphasise the blackness of the characters they were designed to contain. Suicide here was an impossibility. You could suffer in a cell like this for decades I discovered.

My escort returned and looked at me through the grill with the same evil black eyes. Accompanying him was a bald-headed man in a white uniform sniggering to himself. The man, a convict, dealt out food in the hospital wing. The prison officer, who was enjoying the situation as much as the convict, handed me a "plastic" suit with short sleeves and short legs and some slippers with heels like clogs.

"Put this on" he ordered.

After I had changed the convict grabbed my prison clothes and asked me if I would like something to read. I nodded my head, the prison officer locked my cell door and both he and the convict disappeared down the passage. The minutes ticked by then the man in white and the prison officer returned. The former had a book in his hand and this he slipped through the grill. I gratefully accepted it.

The book was the bible.

After I had absorbed that shock I said to the bald-headed convict in a whisper: "I'm not going to be stuck here forever am I?"

The prison officer had stuck my main charge, attempt to endanger life, on my cell door and I hoped that one or the other might know what sort of sentence it was likely to carry. The bald-headed convict simply said, with a hint of menace in his voice:

"You should not have done what you did."

The prison officer couldn't conceal his delight at this and his face lit up in a broad evil smile. He and the convict then abruptly turned away from my cell door and marched down the passage giving vent to a loud cackling underlying the terrible fate awaiting me.

I sat down on the cold floor in a corner of the cell and opened the bible: "In the beginning God created the heavens and the earth. The earth was without form and void and darkness was upon the face of the deep..." I thought of Cardiff Jail hospital wing, of the primeval atmosphere of the place, of the total meaninglessness that surrounded me. Evil reigned supreme in this new world and even the bible was a joke. Despite its magnificence it offered no consolation for the true nature of my predicament. I sat in a heap on the floor and contemplated my four walls. Down the passage I heard snorts as of caged animals. Between the snorting maniacal laughter would break forth. A prisoner who was going mad in his cell suddenly gave vent to a unearthly screaming. I absorbed these sounds with horror.

I rose and started to move about my cell distractedly as if by constant movement I could throw off my increasing claustrophobia. I walked in small circles my slippers clattering on the hard floor. The fear that there might never be an escape from these four walls was what principally induced the claustrophobia. As I thought about my dungeon the claustrophobia grew until I felt as if I was suffocating like a man trapped in a submarine alone at the bottom of the sea. I started to bang frantically on the wall with my fists. Realising the futility of the exercise I sat down on the mattress and pulled a blanket tightly round myself. Then I started to laugh hysterically and an answering laugh came to me from down the passage.

At that point Mr Griffiths words came back to me: "You must stop protecting your friends. Think what bastards they have been." So I thought of all their unpleasant behaviour towards me, not just of the conspiracy presumably masterminded by Enid to get me locked up in perpetuity but of the mockery I had endured in other ways, things I hadn't thought about before. Suddenly I started to cry. The horror of my situation meant that what I could have faced before had now reduced me to tears. Was Mr Griffiths being deliberately brutal in sending me to this nightmare with no words of reassurance about how long I would do? Did he hope for a reaction, one that would make me condemn my friends along the lines indicated in "Carmarthen General Hospital".

After about ten minutes I heard a sound at the door of my cell and tearfully looked up. Through the grill I noticed a face looking at me; I recognised the piercing eyes of the doctor. He I saw was my only hope. At that moment he might have been a god for like a god he now ruled my destiny. The door was opened and a prison officer gave me a blue dressing gown to put on. I accompanied the doctor to the doorway of his richly upholstered study at the end of the passage; the prison officer followed behind.

"What's the matter young lad?" enquired the doctor.

The tone of his voice was honeyed and cajoling like Enid's had been and I was immediately put on my guard. Authority was only nice to you if it wanted information out of you. I said:

"All my friends are against me." Only two or three were I knew but it felt as if it was all at that moment. And my voice was little more than a squeak.

"How are they against you?" asked the doctor in the same cajoling voice as if he wanted to find out, not about the sordid behaviour of people towards me but about my mind as if there lurked some hideous secrets in its depths.

Nothing in my defence would be accepted I knew so I decided to say what Mr Griffiths and everyone in "Carmarthen General Hospital" were urging me to say: "My friends used to tease me in public over my nose."

The doctor became interested in the charges I faced though I refused to admit to desire to kill which would have been an unfair condemnation of myself. I was asked about Enid.

"She was evil" I replied.

"In what way was she evil?"

She mocked me about my sexual performance." I might better have instanced her lies, particularly those that had placed me in this present hell. But the doctor was not interested in Enid's bad points, only in protecting her and condemning me leading me to assume he must be the prosecution psychiatrist though I was to see just about all psychiatrists were for the prosecution. And he asked me if in fact I had been to bed with her.

"Yes" I replied.

"What form of contraception did you use?"

"She used a diaphragm."

At that point he changed tack and asked:

"Did you use a gun?"

Though it had not been taken with anything terribly sinister in mind I replied that I had used a shotgun.

"How many cartridges did you have in your pocket? Two or three?"

"Thirteen" I replied.

The number was in fact nineteen. But hearing the number thirteen he might have queried it though I did not mention my farfetched idea of getting the police to shoot me, the reason.

The prison officer was called and I was led back to my cell. I had found it a tremendous relief to be momentarily let out of it but once I had returned the dressing gown and the cell door had shut behind me I became ever more conscious of the barrenness and isolation of my four walls.

A few minutes later I heard the doctor's voice outside my cell door. He was talking to a prison officer, no doubt deliberately in earshot of me, saying that a Dr. Capstick, an outside doctor, could give a second opinion.

That night I lay down on my foam mattress and tried to get to sleep. The inner despair and desolation I felt was like nothing I had known. During the course of the night I started awake several times prompted by the pernicious lies in the police statements. The total amount of sleep I got was very little and by the time the lights came on at six o'clock I was wide awake.

At seven the prison officers came on duty and it was a relief to hear their movements and the life they generated. A little later a prison officer unlocked my cell door for slopping out and I felt a real sense of exhilaration as I stepped into the passage and put on the slippers that had been taken from me after my interview with the doctor the previous evening.

As I put them on I wondered why they had been taken away from me the previous evening. I knew that they made a noise so that if you kicked the skirting board in anger your venom would be easily noticed by the prison officers. I contemplated this all the way to the sluice and back again. At my cell door I was again ordered to take off my slippers. A little later I was let out to shave. The prison officers had assembled with razors near the latrines and as I walked down the passage I started to kick at the skirting board in a way to suggest I was angry in line with the defence proposed by Mr Griffiths. A prison officer asked me what the matter was. "I feel annoyed" I said though I was too despondent to be angry. Suddenly three prison officers hastened towards me and led me back to my cell. There they made me sit on the floor. Another prison officer appeared with a sphygmomanometer and my blood pressure was measured. It proved to be normal and my action failed to produce significant results.

But at breakfast time I was brought some largactil which I had been prescribed the previous night. It was an anti-hallucinogen or major tranquilliser and had the effect of a chemical strait jacket on me rather than a sedative and was to prove the start of another form of agony. I started to hyperventilate and I was subject to continuous bodily twitches and movements particularly of the feet. It also had the effect of knocking out of me any remaining life making me less resistant to interrogation.

My breakfast was brought to my cell. It consisted of a bowl of porridge without the luxury of sugar or milk and unused to such austerity and having lost my appetite I left it uneaten.

Later that morning a prison officer said that Dr. P. whom I guessed was the prison doctor, wanted to speak to me. The dressing gown was brought and I was escorted to his study. The prison officer remained outside. Dr. P. asked me to tell him about the girl, Enid.

"There's nothing to tell" I replied.

"Was she a witch?"

I was shocked by the suggestion and replied: "No."

"Was she the most evil woman in the world?"

"No."

He must have thought I thought of Enid as a supernatural incarnation of evil. Rubbish. I had been brainwashed to believe the supernatural did not exist and this sounded terrifying. Because he had seen me in tears the previous evening he had made a snap decision that I must be mad without properly analysing why I was in tears. In a minute or two he had dismissed me from his study and told everyone of importance over the phone that I was clearly mad. Now I had contradicted his opinion. As I had not given the answers he wanted the interview was terminated and the prison officer was called to take me back to my cell.

For the rest of the morning I wandered about my cell totally sick with worry. I had gathered a blanket about my shoulders for comfort and as I walked I went over everything in my mind that had been said in the study that morning. The effect of my fretting was to make me deeply depressed.

Sometime that morning Dr. Pears phoned up Dr. P. offering me a bed in Exe Vale. There in an outside hospital I would at least have had a relative amount of freedom and after a sensible psychiatric report had been made could have been released. Dr. P. replied to Dr. Pears offer of help that I was "highly dangerous". The irony was that I had not been at all violent as far as he could see. This was an assumption based purely on having noted my main charge. Dr. Pears didn't want to have anything more to do with me after that. Indeed in keeping me in prison Dr. P. knew he had a better chance of breaking me. But if breaking people was policy amongst many doctors it did not necessarily get the truth out of you. It just got what the doctor wanted to hear, usually something very different.

After a long morning lunch came. It was brought to me on a plastic plate and consisted of cabbage, heart and potato skins burned to a crisp. Because my meal was so unappetising and because I still had no appetite I again left it uneaten.

That afternoon Dr. Capstick passed my cell door. He took upon himself the liberty of walking through the hospital wing where he could see the conditions of the prisoners for himself. He obviously knew a little of what he was about. Unfortunately I didn't know what I was about at that moment. I was not in a fit state to defend myself or state my case properly.

A short while later Dr. P. came to my cell door and unlocked it. A prison officer as usual gave me a blue dressing gown to put on, and Dr. P. led me to the end of the passage.

"You tell the doctor that you thought Enid was the devil and you will go to his hospital" he said. I later found out that Dr. P. had written several books and that he had a name to preserve which unfortunately meant proving I was mad, but while I still had my wits about me I had no intention of coming out with something like that which would have been getting things out of all proportion. But I did think that the doctors wanted violence which even if untrue might guarantee me a bed.

I was let into the interview room. It was modern and comfortable and most of the solicitors, barristers and doctors who visited the prison never saw what the real conditions for prisoners were like. The room was well-lit and had a big window with bars on it that looked onto a wide lawn. Dr. Capstick was seated in a chair behind a desk with some writing paper in front of him. I sat down in the chair opposite him. Then in a soothing gentle voice he asked me my name and age and the age of the girl in question before inviting me to talk about myself. I began with the teasing over the nose but he cut me short seeing it was a silly explanation so I referred to the retrogressive nose refinements instead. Dr. Capstick surmised that that might have caused anger but as I spoke it became apparent that in fact it was depression I had felt. That might have explained my wanting to draw attention to myself but not the charges I faced. In desperation I realised that play-acting was all that was left to me. So when I launched into my story I was only too eager to follow any cues given and kept exaggerating my feelings. For example I said that after the second retrogressive nose refinement I was "screaming" instead of just crying. I said my motive for picking up the gun was revenge though I had not felt any desire for revenge and that was nonsense. I just hoped he might diagnose me as over the brink of madness, a qualification to go to his hospital I believed. When I spoke of Enid's slanders I called her evil in the process reiterating the word as I saw the doctors interest increase. But I grossly over-emphasised the malice and underplayed the depression. I said it was the law of the jungle and that Enid was "shiny and bright on the outside but rotten inside." I had to stand up and mime what happened on the landing when I went up to Enid's room with the gun. I described the trap though was too close to things to have been able to use the word and I knew no one would brook any criticism of Enid. My father had said that my action was attention seeking and that was what I assumed, wrongly, that Dr. E.'s report had said and if I had known that I had just been written off I would never have dreamed of mentioning any mythical violence. I mentioned my wanting to get the gun three days in a row but the truth was that I had just been determined to get attention and there was nothing sinister in it. And it was only when I was drunk. My only mercy was that it was accepted I did not have murder on the brain. As Dr. Capstick picked up his papers and rose he said:

"I may see you again." I didn't know whether his words boded hope but certainly I was not going to be offered a bed in his hospital.

At four o'clock that afternoon my "evening " meal was brought to my cell. The prison officer who brought it was the same one who had brought the previous meals. As usual I was unable to eat and when he returned and saw the plate of untouched food he accused me of malingering and said he would "get" me.

That night the worst depression of my life settled over me. With the departure of Dr. Capstick I also saw the departure of any viable hope of release and if I had been depressed the previous evening I was now totally frantic. I didn't give a fig about Enid; I just wanted her totally out of my life. Barbara had also disappeared from my mind. My looks did not seem of importance. Only my parents mattered. I needed protectors and they rose up in the shape of my parents. The world had become a horrible and frightening place. I could only trust two people, my mother and my father. Though I had grown away from my mother and father in late adolescence now I had lost everything they were everything. In a corner of my cell I discovered a sheet of prison letterhead and after I had managed to get hold of a pen I wrote them the most desperate letter of my life. I spoke of how many lies had been told, of how I had been framed and made out to be an ogre but that they alone knew the truth, that I was good. I said I wanted to see them one last time.

When I slopped out the following morning I was allowed to mingle with the other prisoners. The latrines were crowded and stunk of urine and excrement some of which had splashed on the floor. A steamy mass of urine, excrement and toilet paper swirled about in the sluice. Amongst the prisoners in the crowd was a man who had covered himself in his own excrement even rubbing it into his hair whilst in a state of nervous breakdown in his cell. Seeing such a thing filled me with a horror that stayed with me all the way back to my cell.

At breakfast I was allowed to go and collect my meal from the hatch at the end of the corridor. A line of prisoners had formed, some with stories to justify that impression of caged destructive evil that I had gained on my arrival. Up front in a position to receive the largest helpings was a man in a "tracksuit" indicating he was on a murder charge. He was about six feet eight tall and of broad build; he was perfectly calm and collected. No one questioned his position of dominance and he didn't have to throw his tremendous weight about to prove it. He was deeply respected by the prisoners and the prison officers alike; not a soul dared cross him. Further down was a man in a plastic suit. His arms and legs were covered in a massive overgrowth of hair. He looked like a cross between a gorilla and a human being and was in a padded cell. He was insane with grief and was standing just in front of the medicine trolley where prisoners received their largactil in tears. Behind him were those in strip cells, the potential suicides, the lowest of the low. They too were in a desperate state. One later swallowed a needle he managed to get hold of. I took my place amongst the potential suicides.

142

When my turn came to receive my breakfast the man in white gave me a tiny dollop of everything even though I was beginning to recover my appetite. The rest he kept for himself. He fed like a king on all the juicy morsels left over.

Back in my cell I wondered: "Was I condemned to this jungle for the rest of my days?" The thought of a lifelong hell in such a place worked on my mind most horribly all that morning. It was like being in a war. But you at least had hope of coming out of a war, of something coming out of it. My chances of coming out of this, of anything coming out of it, seemed nil. No one who could help seemed remotely interested in rescuing me from my nightmare and seeing no hole whatsoever in the opposition against me I did not see how I could escape my fate. I had always thought martyrdom senseless particularly for the poor victim. Now my life was to be needlessly sacrificed.

That afternoon I saw my parents for a fifteen minute visit, the maximum time allowed. We met in the interview room and a prison officer was present. I was dressed in my plastic suit, my slippers and my blue dressing gown.

They sat down at one end of the table, I at the other. The prison officer sat in a corner of the room guarding the seconds. I tried to ignore him and concentrate on my parents. I wanted to be close to them as possible and the table between us was like a great divide. At least I was able to hold my mother's hand. But I knew that all too soon authority would come between us and the prison officer, ruled by his watch, would cold-bloodedly separate us. And I said: "Mum! Dad! Oh my God!" "Never mind my darling" said my mother squeezing my hand tightly. After a pause my father said: "I don't know what to say." "What about Mr Griffiths?" I asked as if he might still be able to help. "He said they are still trying to find you a bed" replied my mother. Even now I had a very faint hope that I would escape to the relative freedom of a hospital. The word hospital conjured up visions of the psychiatric unit in "Carmarthen General Hospital" where the nurses, both male and female, were like angels in comparison with the prison officers. Common sense for the most part belied any real hope that a return to such a place was now a possibility and I said with a trace of despair: "I saw a Dr. Capstick yesterday but nothing came of it. Dr. P. isn't much help either." I went onto discuss the cats at home and my sister. They too had assumed enormous significance for me. I felt them to be an essential part of what I had lost.

All too soon the prison officer rose from his seat and said that my time was up. I drew myself away from my parents with as much dignity as I could muster and was led back to my cell.

On the Thursday the assistant chaplain paid me a visit. He was young and friendly and even sat down next to me on the floor

143

of my cell. He asked me how I felt and I explained I did not feel too happy. He said he had worked in a mental hospital before he became ordained and seemed to have more understanding than most. And though he had six hundred lost sheep to minister to he was to devote plenty of time to me. He was the first person in prison I liked. Before he left he gave me a book on Christianity which I had a quick look through.

The next Monday I shaved and bathed. I was given some prison clothes to change into. I had an early breakfast which consisted of a boiled egg and a slice of bread before being escorted to the reception area. There I changed from my prison clothes into civvies for the trip to Abaraeron Magistrates Court. I was handcuffed to a prison officer and my holdall was placed in the boot of a waiting taxi. Wedged in the back between two prison officers I commenced the long journey to Abaraeron.

At the magistrates court I met Mr Griffiths and my parents in a room in the court building. My parents had seen me everyday except Sunday since their first prison visit. In the gallery through the door I noticed the chaplain of Lampeter University and the president of the students union who both gave me encouraging smiles. I also noticed the female reporter. Back in the room Mr Griffiths said:

"We're trying to find you a bed."

I was confused as to why there was so much talk about finding me a bed and so much difficulty in obtaining one. What I did not know was that Dr. P. was insisting on sending me to a closed hospital under section 60/65 of the Mental Health Act. A closed hospital was a secure as any prison in the British Isles. In addition the section 65 meant I could be detained in such a place for the rest of my natural life; dangerous killers and rapists were sent to such places. I had simply been led to expect I would be going to a place like the psychiatric unit at "Carmarthen General Hospital". The whole thing was a cruel joke.

I still had some wits about me and knew the constant isolation combined with the knowledge of having been framed was what made me so depressed. So I asked Mr Griffiths when I would be let out amongst the other prisoners. He didn't reply and I didn't know that Dr. P. would on no account let me leave the hospital wing. There was a reasonably comfortable dormitory just above the passage which I knew nothing about and where I could have been perfectly happy. But the passage in which I was held was deliberately macabre and the isolation combined with the horror was it seemed designed to break you. While I remained in isolation I became ever more malleable and liable to make statements that would ensure I was sent to a prison hospital.

I was led into the court room. The hearing was a mere formality and I was remanded in custody for another week. Even the bringing of the holdall was a cruel joke for I stood no real prospect of being released to a hospital and it was just one way of building up my hopes before dashing them. I remained calm and collected. I was not allowed to speak to my parents again so went outside and sat in the taxi. A prison officer kindly lent me the Sun to read and I was reasonably happy and buoyant while I read it. Reading a newspaper was not something I was allowed to do in jail. I also remained calm during the long journey back to Cardiff Jail. But once in the hospital wing the reality of the situation hit me again. The man in white refused me my supper, I had missed out on lunch and the all-round deprivation of food, daylight and emotional warmth all conspired to destroy me.

That Tuesday I saw Dr. P. again but only after I had pestered him to allow me a word. All I wanted was a sign of reassurance but he only had one plan, to send me to a closed hospital and to give me reassurance at this stage would only have succeeded in defeating his object as I would not then have been prone to self-condemnation. The interview that ensued was to become typical. Dr. P. asked me if I heard voices, if I thought people were plotting against me and if Enid was the devil. Each time I answered truthfully that I did not hear voices and that I did not think Enid was the devil the interview would be terminated. I never said I thought there was a conspiracy for I knew he would just say I was hallucinating. The interview as always lasted less than a minute and I left the study feeling much worse.

Over the next few weeks I continued to see Dr. P. for a minute a day excepting weekends. I still had not received any reassurance from him. Everytime I walked into the study I hoped for reassurance. Indeed the study had a fatal fascination. But he had made up his mind and nothing would change it. I was knocking my head against a brick wall and these interviews could do only one thing. They gave me ample opportunity to unfairly condemn myself. Self-condemnation was almost unavoidable for Dr. P. would set traps and only by the utmost care and control was I able to avoid them. I did very rarely make statements for the sake of making them. However I was slowly getting a picture of what he wanted me to say by noting the questions he asked. I was greatly worried for not only was the picture far from the truth, it was damning. I fully saw the dangerous ideas he had about me but what I had to say was getting beyond my control. As there are usually only prosecution psychiatrists truth and justice has virtually nothing to do with it.

After a month in Cardiff Jail during a visit from my mother I asked what was happening. She said that she could not get hold of Mr Griffiths. His unavailability was obviously due to the fact that he had no further words of hope to offer my parents. My distress became obvious and the prison officer in the room said:

"If you can't do the time don't commit the crime."

That was the view of many but certain people had determined I was guilty before I had been tried and matters were far more complex than that. I never set out to commit a crime and I had been framed. My mother and I spoke about generalities then I exclaimed:

"Well, Dr.Capstick was a waste of time. Mr Griffiths was a waste of time. In fact they're all a waste of time."

I was losing faith in everyone except my parents. I left my mother that day believing my parents were all I had left.

Meanwhile the man in white was continuing his war of attrition and now had a deliberate policy of starving me. Invariably I got tiny helpings at meal times and at supper when he came round with the rock cakes he would miss my cell. When I went to court all I was allowed for the day was the one compulsory boiled egg. I dreamt of food. My hunger was with me day and night. I had felt hungry at school on occasions but this was real hunger. He had elected to come to the hospital wing to gloat and that was what he was doing. I was being viewed as a freak.

The man in the cell opposite me said: "I don't like what they are doing to you." He got a cleaner to give me a Mars bar. The man had a very quick temper and an even quicker fist but at least he had a good heart.

The next Monday I returned as usual to Abaraeron Magistrates Court with my holdall of clothes. Deep down knew I would as usual return to Cardiff Jail at the end of the day. But I had another misfortune in store for me that day for Mr Griffiths had absented himself from the hearing. Someone came up to me in the waiting room and said he was standing in for Mr Griffiths. I thought that now was the right moment to glean some true facts about my case and I whispered to the man:

"How long will I do?"

The man didn't reply.

"Will I do life?"

He just turned his head away as if he couldn't bring himself to tell me the terrible truth of the situation.

I assumed from there on that I would do life. At best life might mean thirty years. I thought but thirty years might as well have been a thousand years. When I got out my parents would be dead and I would be something approaching an old man. I had hardly left school. I had been full of ideals. Now I had lost everything. The vision of my life reduced to meaninglessness, the belief that there was no light at the end of the tunnel was too much to bear. With the disappearance of Mr Griffiths I had seen the disappearance of all hope. I was overcome by an uncontrollable shaking.

As I walked into the court room it was obvious to everyone that I had ceased to be the person I was. My twitching and shaking was wrongly interpreted as an admission of guilt as if I had been found out. I was just totally broken. On seeing me the chaplain of Lampeter University turned away in disgust. Though he was a chaplain he was also flesh and blood and though he and the president of the students union did attend future hearings it was only as a way of getting information for the university about me and neither of them showed any encouragement or interest in me anymore.

The hearing ended and I was taken to the waiting taxi. I could not have read the newspaper now even if I had tried. On the way back to Cardiff Jail I twitched continuously between the two prison officers on either side of me.

That night I decided it would be in my interests to feign madness. I was halfway along the road to being driven mad anyway. A prisoner had told me that in a hospital I would be able to have two hourly visits a day rather than the half hour per fortnight I would be allowed if I was given a prison sentence. I felt totally wretched about the prospect of doing life in a prison and doing life in a closed hospital. But in the end a closed hospital seemed the better of the two evils and as I stood in the medicine queue on future occasions I would deliberately make a long face and start to cry in front of the prison officers so that it would seem I was not strong enough for prison and that I was sufficiently disturbed to warrant a hospital place.

The pressure on me was continuing to mount and I was still being starved, something that worried my mother. On a visit with my father she handed me a packet of almond slices and I slipped them under the elastic of my shorts out of sight of the supervising officer who was sitting in a chair outside the room. Other remand prisoners were allowed food to be brought in. As I was in a strip cell I was denied such privileges. This was arguably to prevent me obtaining the means to commit suicide. I could never work out how you could commit suicide with an almond slice.

At the end of the visit the prison officer who had accused me of malingering came and escorted me back to my cell. As I removed my dressing gown at my cell door he turned and said:

"Okay, what have you got hidden away?"

"Nothing" I stammered.

"I'm no fool. What have you go hidden away?"

"Nothing."

"Hold up your arms."

I held my arms up and the almond slices remained safely concealed underneath the elastic of my shorts. The prison officer looked very puzzled. Then after reflecting for a bit, he lifted up my top. The almond slices were clearly in evidence.

"I told you I would get you" he said. He took the almond slices and ordered me into my strip cell locking the door. I heard him instruct another prison officer to return the almond slices to my parents. He returned to my cell and said through the bars:

"If ever I catch you smuggling in this prison again there will be a headline: Vicar Caught Smuggling and your father's name will be dirt."

My father had not himself been involved in "smuggling" and my mother had simply been concerned over the way I was getting nothing to eat. It was devastating how authority was not just out to condemn me but my parents as well.

One mercy was that a murderer helping in the hospital wing started to surreptitiously slip hard boiled eggs and biscuits to me through my grill after that. The murderer was the kindest and most pleasant individual there and his example proved that you don't necessarily have to be mad or bad to be a murderer. But he had come on the scene too late to be of any great assistance for I had already been pressurised into completely condemning myself.

At about this time Mr Griffiths handed over my case to a Mrs Matthews in Cardiff. He had told my parents that the distance was too great for him to travel and that a woman might have a better understanding of me. Probably he had just completely given up on me. He had therefore handed over my case to solicitors experienced in matters of murder and attempted murder for I was being treated as an attempted murderer. A tragic mistake.

I had been in solitary confinement for six weeks and having wandered between abject despair and faint hope, hope as if put there to torment me, Dr. P. broke the last of my resistance. He had kept me at a pitch of anxiety, desperation, even terror. I had withstood it all this time. Then I snapped.

It happened like this. I buttonholed Dr. P. as he walked past my cell door, the blue dressing gown was brought, and I ended up in his study, this time in tears. He usually waited for such a moment before he spoke to a patient, a moment when the patient was likely to be most malleable and suggestible. On this occasion I was allowed to sit down in a chair in the study and he stood over me. Going off on his usual track he asked of Enid:

"Was she the devil?"

"No" I replied between sobs.

"Was she a witch?"

"No."

"Was she Lucifer?"

Still tearful and wondering what other answer I could give to such questions other than "No" I paused.

"Was she Lucifer?" the question came again.

I looked up at my inquisitor then down at my knees and said: "Yes." I had not given that answer because I remotely believed it to be true. The idea to me was entirely ridiculous. But I had given the answer I knew Dr. P. wanted to hear. I had wanted to halt the protracted nightmare and I hoped that if I said what he wanted me to say my case would be dealt with sooner. However in that moment of weakness I knew I had made a terrible mistake. But had I not, the torture would have continued indefinitely.

Dr. P. was immediately on the phone but although I didn't fully realise it, at the other end of the line was Broadmoor.

CHAPTER 11
FATE SEALED.

The day after the fatal interrogation with Dr. P., my barrister, Mr G. W., visited me for the first time obviously having been informed that the interrogations were over. Accompanying him were a Mr Evans who was an assistant to Mrs Matthews, and a Law student. It was obvious to me that Dr. P. must have told Mr G. W. the result of the previous day's interrogation and as a consequence my defence lawyers now thought of me as a dangerously sick proposition. Before I entered the interview room I determined to set the picture straight but appreciating on entering, that Mr G. W. had swallowed everything that Dr. P. had said, I burst into tears instead.

I sat down and my barrister produced some papers which he started to go through. His manner was of efficiency and self-assuredness. But he had read the statements to the police and it was apparent from his voice that he wasn't even going to try and defend the apparently indefensible. He said:

"The idea is to send you to Rampton or Broadmoor. You could do a few weeks there or very many years."

By the way he spoke I assumed I would have to spend very many years in a psychiatric prison. I wanted to scrap the psychiatric option now that I knew what it entailed but my lawyers already regarded me as a dangerous lunatic.

"I have worked with Dr. P. for many years and I trust him to be an honourable man." He spoke to me as if my honour was in doubt.I found such talk of honour a total irony. During my time in "Carmarthen General Hospital" I had been the only one to show any honour. I could even have got off the hook had I desired. But somehow all the perjurers came across as honourable, as having loyally done their duty to the state. And I came across as devious and underhand.

I went on to try and discount some of what Dr. P. had got me to say under psychological torture, notably the notion that Enid was the devil. Mr G. W. replied:

"You did think that she was the devil."

I now stood no chance of a fair trial. My counsel had joined the ranks of the opposition and the big guns on both sides were ranged against me. The interview ended. Mr G. W., Mr Evans and the law student rose and left and I decided there was nothing left but to play along with everyone.

I wondered why Mrs Matthews had not been to see me. I found out that she had been too frightened to come because Dr. P. had said that I was highly dangerous and that as she was a woman I might attack her if she visited me. As well as being sheer nonsense such words made for a bad start. In order to try and stem the growing paranoia (or was it just evil?) of authority my father visited my solicitors offices and said to Mr Evans that he did not think I was a schizophrenic as Dr. P. was trying to make out. It was clear that my solicitors were totally under the power of Dr. P. and just accepted whatever he said. When my father pointed out the contradictory opinion of the first psychiatric report he just retorted that I had "pulled the wool over their eyes." My defence was working hand in glove with the prosecution psychiatrist.

My mother telephoned MIND about my conditions. They in turn wanted to interview me but the prison authorities turned down their request. My father saw his MP who was entirely sympathetic and even suggested an arrangement whereby I remain at home not venturing beyond the garden. Dr. P. would have none of it. The MP got in touch with the Chief Constable of Devon and Cornwall who suggested bail. The suggestion was turned down. My father wrote to the prison governor. The letter was just passed on to Dr. P. who was in turn infuriated and stormed over to my cell angrily shaking the bars. He didn't like being contradicted. A day or two later Mrs Matthews received a letter from Dr. P. saying that if there were any more irritations he would bring legal pressure to bear against my parents. She informed my parents that they were doing terrible damage to my case. My father, a man of the cloth, stood to be branded a liar, and my parents, my natural protectors, silenced.

Dr. Capstick appeared on the scene again as he said he might do. A little before the interview I had asked Dr. P. how long I would do in hospital and he had said eighteen months to two years in a closed hospital and a year in an open hospital but though I didn't fully believe him I had settled down so decided to play along and when I sat down said that Enid was a witch. Dr. Capstick shook his head dismissing that as rubbish which it was. Mrs Matthews assistant had indicated that at that stage I would have done eight years in prison which didn't bother me but at that stage it seemed I would be more likely to obtain justice taking the psychiatric option. Though Dr. Capstick hinted at bail I did not follow it up. But at the end of the day he did not offer me a bed in his hospital. Rescue appeared out of the question now. And I tended to think in terms of doing life.

The day after, as I shaved, the man in the tracksuit started to chat to me saying: "You're putting on a good act." In desperation I had as seen been driven to act a certain amount but that was not because I was bad. It was because I couldn't stand the torture. The man in the tracksuit had previous experience of prison. He knew the ropes and what to expect. On questioning him it emerged that he was able to forget about his family whom he knew he would never see again. When he committed his crime he knew how much time he would do and that he was capable of doing it. I hadn't planned or

151

remotely anticipated what had happened to me. I had only set out to create a stir, not to commit murder. I hadn't anticipated having to spend decades inside when I picked up the gun, and unlike this man could not face that.

A day or two later a prison officer appeared at my cell door and said to me through the grill that a doctor had come to take me away.I was overjoyed at such unexpected news and when the cell door was opened I put on my dressing gown with enthusiasm. But having trusted Dr. Capstick I was now frightened of being let down again and I determined that the matter be finalised. That meant going to a hospital and I didn't envisage Rampton or Broadmoor but an ordinary psychiatric hospital with a closed ward where, after a spell, I would be discharged.

So when I entered the interview room I deliberately said out loud of Enid in what was a snap decision:

"She's evil."

I believed that hostility was what the doctors wanted and that such a statement would get me a bed and avoid an unfairly long sentence. The doctor who was sitting behind the desk, asked if I was sure I still felt that adding that he was a Dr. Tidmarsh from Broadmoor. I was taken aback at the discovery that I was talking to a Broadmoor doctor but I didn't know how I could retract what I had said. I had heard that Broadmoor was more comfortable than most prisons but I assumed it was such just to make life bearable for people who would never see daylight again and nothing could truly make me want to go there. After I had sat down Dr. Tidmarsh said:

"I have copied out a report made by Dr. P.. I expect you have been through the story many times before so I won't ask you to go through it again."

I realised he had accepted for the most part what Dr. P. had said though he did reject the theory that it was the teasing in public over my nose that was responsible. And he asked me if the nose operation was mentioned on the radio. I said it wasn't. He started to read out the psychiatric report that he had just copied. All the things that I had been obliged to say under torture, notably the allegation that I thought Enid the devil, came out. At that point I tried to stop him and deny that claim. He simply said: "You told Dr. P. you did." I knew that was the end of the matter though all I had ever done was say yes after having said no fifty times to the question as to whether she was Lucifer. I did later gather that Dr. Tidmarsh did write I was suffering from no florid delusions. During the reading of the report all the damaging lies in the police statements were brought up including John's lie about premeditated attempted murder. I denied this but Dr. Tidmarsh said: "You told your friend that you did", utter rubbish. Towards the end of the report I became even more worried for it had been written that I had a "mission to kill Enid." Absolute rubbish. Had I wanted to kill Enid I had had thousands of opportunities and simply would have done so and been treated much less harshly.

I was asked what punishment I thought she deserved. I stupidly said: "She should have her face smashed in." She had after all framed me for life. Dr.Tidmarsh replied that with drink inside I would be homicidal. I was never homicidal even with alcohol inside me. I knew that what was written claimed I was not only completely out of touch with reality but highly dangerous. Dr. Tidmarsh had happily swallowed the lot. If there had been liars the only liar was deemed to be me, the most honest of the lot. Dr. Tidmarsh was completely ignorant of the fact that I was upset precisely by the dangerous ideas of psychiatrists who were graded on how evil they could be in their words. And he along with Dr. H. had set out to get me convicted of all the worst charges I faced. No mention was made of Enid's lies even though I mentioned them to the doctors. I later gathered rightly or wrongly that they had made out I just imagined them. Enid had emerged from the whole business as a spotless angel, I, a deluded monster. I now knew what was meant by the phrase: Trial By Psychiatrist. I anticipated D.Tidmarsh's final remark:

"You are very sick indeed. I will put an order into the court right away."

When I returned to my cell it was with a heaviness of heart. I had believed in wisdom, truth and justice, particularly of the British kind. But my whole life had ended in a miscarriage of justice. I had never really stood a chance. Strength combined with aggression had as always won the day. But it was as if for the moment I could do no more.

I found out that the bald-headed man in white had left the hospital wing. I gathered he had been sacked. No doubt he had started to tread on the toes of authority. It should have been a happy moment and the man's replacement was far more congenial, but he had done his bit towards destroying me and his disappearance at this stage was a hardly a blessing.

Shortly after it had been determined I was going to Broadmoor I was moved out of my strip cell into a furnished cell. Everything necessary to condemn me had been said therefore if I committed suicide it would now be attributed to mental illness and not to any fault of the authorities. The furnished cell gave me more opportunity to commit suicide than a strip cell. But I was slightly happier there even though my fate was sealed. I had a desk to write on, a bed with sheets, pillow, blankets, coverlet and a chair. Compared with the strip cell it was very comfortable. I was also entitled to more privileges. These included being allowed a radio and having sweets, food and soft drinks brought in from outside. I was also allowed to wear prison clothes and thus I could take half an hours exercise a day.

I informed a prison officer peering through the grill that I was destined for Broadmoor. It wasn't a widely known fact in the hospital wing and it was assumed I was just imagining things. I repeated that I was going to Broadmoor. The prison officer still refused to believe me. I told other prison officers of the decision to send me to Broadmoor. My words were met with incredulity. It was inconceivable to most that I should be going to Broadmoor for I had not been at all violent or abusive in prison. But my protestations and then a word from someone in the know finally convinced them.

After that I was faced with continuous harassment. For example as I was walking round the exercise yard one day I placed my hand on a spot on my head that had been numbed by the largactil when the supervising officer barked at me to come over. I was seized by the collar and rudely led indoors back to my cell. The prison officers thought of me as a freak now that I was going to Broadmoor. As far as they could understand only the worst cases went to Broadmoor so they concluded that I must be a monster. Even the shuffling of my feet which only started when I was put on drugs was blamed on something abnormal in my psychological make-up. The prison officer who had accused me   of malingering on the other hand became very pleasant.

A prison officer passing through the hospital wing stopped at my cell and started to chat through the grill. I told him that I was destined for Broadmoor and said that I had been told it was a holiday camp for a prison officer in authority had said that to me to try and reassure me. The prison officer exclaimed out loud: "On no. I used to live near Broadmoor. I was shown round the hospital. It's a terrible place." Perhaps unintentionally, by the time he left, I had a vision of Broadmoor as a walled fortress, of patients locked in dark little dungeons, some chained to the walls. I imagined them possessed by devils ready to punch, scratch or bite any living thing in sight. I had seen films like the Nuns Story where lunatics were so depicted and I had had no one to disillusion me. It was a forbidding thought.

When I was next in the exercise yard which was a cramped little court yard surrounded by a high wall, I treasured that glimpse of daylight and blue sky which I thought might be my last. I felt the need to savour the fresh air of the exercise yard while it seemed I could. I even felt sorry to leave a column of smoke that I saw rising from a nearby industrial estate. I could almost understand why some prisoners like Jimmy Boyle had lived in fear of being. certified insane.

On the evening before my crown court appearance Mr G. W. , Mr Evans and a second Law student paid me a visit and we all met as usual in the interview room. Once I was settled and comfortable I was shown a few photographs, one of Enid with a cut on her forehead, one of a sapling shredded at the bottom and one of my room at college which was an untidy mess. Then with his usual efficiency and briskness Mr G.W. started to page through the police statements tying up loose ends. If my statement was too harsh on myself and far from a justification it was at least accepted by my barrister. I quoted what Mr Griffiths had said, that it was written for me. Mr G. W. responded: "These are not the words of a simple policeman." The point was that the police's influence was clear and he criticised me for trying to "tailor" the statements. We considered what I should plead guilty to. It was determined I should plead guilty to attempt to commit an indictable offence. Also to causing actual bodily harm though when I had caused the scratch to Enid's forehead I had not deliberately set out to do so. Mr G. W. accepted that when I took Tony's gun I had not meant he shouldn't have it back. So it was decided I would not plead guilty to theft of a shotgun though I would to being in possession of a shotgun without a shotgun certificate. Though the charges did not worry me I was worried that my defence would be insanity. Thus the prosecution witnesses were going to become defence witnesses and most of their slanders were going to be used as so-called evidence of insanity.

I mentioned the side effects of the drugs.I would not have minded the drugs had I felt that they had been helping me but Mr G. W. spoke as if they were the one thing between me and a strait jacket. I did not press the point.

He produced Dr. Capstick's report, a report that greatly shocked me. He did not help matters by saying that I was not in control when I went up to Enid's room with the gun though I had been in as much control and no more dangerous than a car driver. I don't know where he got that from and it might have just been incorrect extrapolation. But the report was not nearly as extreme as Dr. P.'s report and I almost expected the diagnosis of paranoid schizophrenia after my desperate play-acting. However I thought prison a better bet than Broadmoor if the psychiatrists opinions were accepted and I expressed that preference. "You'll probably do longer in prison than in hospital" said Mr G. W.. He said I would do six years in prison taking into account remission, three in Broadmoor. If he was right I would have had no problem in prison or a closed hospital. But always at the forefront of my mind was the fear that if I went to Broadmoor one look at Dr. Tidmarsh's report would ensure I never got out. I believed that whatever was decided in court would bear little relation to how long I was locked up for in a hospital and when my lawyers left I still had nagging doubts.

The next day, after a seemingly endless wait for a taxi, I was driven to Swansea Crown Court secured between two prison officers. The court case was due to start at ten o'clock but we arrived after that hour. I was extremely apprehensive, particularly about what the future held in store for me. My last chance of avoiding going to Broadmoor was just to take my defence into my own hands and blurt out all I thought and felt. But I was nervous that if I did try and do that the law might come down on me even harder for opposing the "expert"witnesses. It was a tricky moment and I didn't feel my lone voice would be heeded.

I was escorted below court into the dungeons where I met Mr G. W. a pretty young female Law student, Mrs Matthews and Dr. P.. The Law student I assumed had been planted there just to prove to the judge that I was not going to attack the first girl in sight after all. Mr Evans was not present.

A little later Mr G. W. presented me with the charge sheet. On top of the list of charges was that of attempt to endanger life. The charge of attempt to commit an indictable offence was not on the sheet. Only the charge of attempt to commit an indictable offence namely to cause grievous bodily harm. As a result of a plea bargain with the prosecution it was agreed that I plead guilty to that rather than the main charge.

I mentioned my doubts about the psychiatric reports. Mr G. W. told me to discuss the matter with Dr. P. Alone in a room I said to him I was deeply unhappy about the psychiatric reports. He replied: "You're the most difficult patient I've had in ten years" and he stormed out of the room. There was nothing I could do at this stage to alter the psychiatrists recommendations. They had little understanding of why I had been in such a terrible state on my admittance to Cardiff Jail hospital wing, namely being framed then put in a dungeon seemingly for life. The chaplain had spoken of Dr. P.'s cruel to be kind approach, but two people out of an intake of fifteen later committed suicide two days in a row because of this approach it seemed. And though Dr. P. may have thought he was helping me in sending me to a hospital, Broadmoor was hardly a blessing.

I was led up some stairs to the dock. From there I faced the judge in his wig and red robes. Immediately in front of me were Mrs Matthews and then the prosecution and my barristers. Behind me in the gallery I noticed my parents and the aggressive detective.

The barristers, impressive in their wigs and gowns, delivered their briefs in turn. Their words were directed towards the judge and I didn't hear very clearly what they had to say. But I did note the attempt of the prosecution counsel to depict me as a dangerous uncontrollable madman.

Dr. P. then stepped into the witness stand, swore an oath before the court and pronounced me insane. The judge had already read a report with the nonsense statement that I was a potential danger to Enid or a substitute.

As the proceedings were taking place in a closed court the "witnesses" were not required to attend so after being pronounced insane I had to plead.

I pleaded not guilty to attempt to endanger life, guilty of attempt to cause grievous bodily harm, not guilty to theft of a shotgun, guilty to causing actual bodily harm and guilty to being in possession of a shotgun without a shotgun certificate. I was perfectly calm when I made my pleas and they were accepted.

Afterwards the judge said that I was to be sent to a special hospital within twenty eight days. He concluded: "I hope you get better soon" and I had no complaints with him. He must have had some heart and there was no trace of vindictiveness in his manner or words. But I still assumed he must only have read Dr. Capstick's report and thus had more hope to offer me than he might otherwise have had.

In the dungeons after the court case I said a courtesy thank you to Mr G. W. who replied that he got "paid for the job" anyway and perhaps sensed I was not at all happy with the outcome. But I wanted things to end on an amicable note.

I was allowed to see my parents though I was divided from them by a glass partition. Words were difficult and it was more cruel than kind to be able to see them but not to be able to touch them. Precisely what they had most feared had happened and at this stage acceptance and quiet was the only thing. In no time at all the supervising prison officer appeared and told us our time was up.

I was handcuffed and led to a waiting taxi. To society it would appear that justice and humanity had been served. How you fared with the law depended on your ability to stand up for yourself or on having good counsel; my counsel had been too influenced by the prosecution case and certainly I had not stood up for myself very well. I felt destined for further punishment rather than treatment. I would have preferred to be in Raskalnikoff's shoes; he was given a limit of seven years in prison after his trial, in Crime and Punishment. Both he and I had suffered in our own way up to our court cases and in the most horrible way. I knew no way out of my suffering. Suffering in many unimaginable forms was a way of life to me now.

Back at Cardiff Jail hospital wing I was moved to the condemned cell where murderers in the past had spent their last days on earth. I now had some notion of what it must be like to be a man condemned to death. My predecessors had only three weeks to wait before they took that short walk to the execution shed and dropped to their deaths. I looked forward to a living death stretching into eternity. Even if I had hoped that the opportunity to see my parents

157

more in hospital would make life more bearable, that thought did not help me now. There was an additional factor in the equation - women. I wondered whether I would not have preferred the rope to a life shut away completely from women.

On my next visit, which was held in the canteen, my mother said that I was on section 60/65 and that I only had eight days to appeal. I was also told that under section 65 I was liable to recall should I ever be released. Both these little details no one had ever told me about. My mother and I considered an appeal. Because of the extreme nature of the psychiatric reports I knew that nothing could come of it.

A day or two later I started to chat again to the man in the tracksuit while I shaved. I went on to tell him I was bound for Broadmoor. He replied: "Oh, I knew someone who went to Broadmoor. He came out a cabbage."

After I had shaved and returned to my cell the man's remark began to play on my mind for I took it literally. Indeed people were turned into cabbages in special hospitals. I thought of McMurphy in One Flew Over The Cuckoo's Nest. He had had his personality and intellect destroyed by a lobotomy and inevitably I believed I was going to have a lobotomy. I recalled the zombies in overalls raking the grounds at St. David's Psychiatric Hospital and wondered whether they had had lobotomies.

That afternoon I became desperate and decided to write Dr. P. a letter denying I was a danger and that I was insane. I hoped that somehow my letter would save me even though I failed to mention the frame-up which along with my conditions had broken me. Sadly I came across as a deceiver rather than the truth, that I was a wronged person. When Dr. P. walked by my cell again I proffered him the letter through the grill. He declined it.

So that night I resigned myself to becoming a cabbage. I thought that it might even be better to be a cabbage and sent home to my parents than caged for life like a wild animal. The night proved to be more peaceful than many.

The next morning my anxiety started up all over again and I nabbed the other prison psychiatrist as he passed my cell door and thrust the letter into his hand. He read the letter, assumed that I was guilty of everything but that I had just been malingering to escape the full punishment and he refused to talk to me when I called him as he passed the door of my cell again. He acted as if he thought I should receive the full harshness of the law.

He then spoke to Dr. P. who simply showed him the police statements and the psychiatric reports and he felt justice had been done but he did not reassure me on the question of the lobotomy which was the crux of the letter.

Even so by the end of the day my fears had died down and when I spoke to the man in the tracksuit again he said: "You'll be out of there in no time" as if it would all be all right. And I should say that Dr. P., appreciating my concerns, did say that I could "sort things out" in Broadmoor.

The next Sunday I attended chapel. Although I never expected religion to offer me a way out it was somehow a consolation and I was amused that the most hardened criminals and the most evil men in the prison also went. Even the bald-headed man attended. There was much enthusiasm during the singing and it was a perfect excuse to escape the cells for an hour. But I was so overcome by the side effects of the drugs that I had difficulty in keeping still and that spoilt the service for me.

A week after my trial I had a nightmare. I was in Broadmoor for a life term and as with many others this made me suicidal. The answer rose in the shape of a suicide chamber. It was a small room with a type of swing bag suspended from the middle of the ceiling out of which blades protruded. The potential suicide would be locked in the chamber and on desperation at his plight would blunder about causing the bag to swing violently. Death would follow. When my turn came, and as death was just about upon me I woke up.

About two weeks after my trial I received a visit from Nick along with my mother. Nick had just returned from a holiday in Jersey with Lorna and had just found out that I was in prison. He had expected me to be freed on the word of a psychiatrist. When I arrived at the canteen the table at which Nick was sitting was littered with Mars bars, flakes, and all manner of sweets. It was one of Nick's occasional displays of generosity and obviously he had been informed of how I had been starved in prison. But I would have preferred him to give useful information rather than assuage my appetite. Little was discussed on this occasion.

However approximately two days later Nick visited me again for a quarter of an hour in the canteen and this time he was alone.

"Can't anything be done? "I asked. "Can't John be persuaded to change his story at all?"

"No" said Nick. After a pause he added: "You are mild. You'll be out of there in no time."

I thought of that as wishful thinking on his part, and as for John; well like Nero, he would fiddle while Rome burned.

I referred to the lie that Enid had told at university which Nick mentioned.

"Enid said that I went up to her room with a knife." My intention in saying this was just to point out that I had been dealing with liars and slanderers all along. Nick replied:

"Well, didn't you?"

Even Nick had been taken in by all the lies now. Now that I was going to Broadmoor, the world, instead of reacting in disbelief at such a prospect, would assume I was both mad and dangerous. People could and would level any slander at me and it would be believed. Ironically if I had been remotely violent or hostile and if I had used one of thousands of chances to kill her I would have been far better off.

"I had to protect Lorna" he said as if to try and mitigate his part in the cover-up cum frame-up but Lorna was never my problem, I liked her and what he could have said to acquit me need never have mentioned Lorna.

I knew it was just hard luck on me. I was just a scapegoat, a bait, a sport, an example of the futility of friendship.

"I will visit you every fortnight in Broadmoor" said Nick.

I did not believe him of course. Promises meant little or nothing. Because I had foundered in the rough sea of living I was now considered of no value. All I could say was that Nick amused me and I would have to stick by people who amused me for I could not expect anymore from people than that.

The end of the visit came and I left for my cell with the knowledge that no one would make any endeavours to rescue me from the prospect of lifelong incarceration.

A day or two later, when I was on association which I was now allowed, I suddenly started to cry. Association which lasted half an hour took place in the dormitory above the passage. The dormitory had big windows that looked over the rest of the prison and the city of Cardiff. There was a black and white television and also a few prisoners to talk to. But I now still felt trapped. My cage was just a little bit bigger this time. The improved surroundings of the dormitory could not and did not distract me from my problems or the fear of permanent incarceration in Broadmoor. One prisoner had known a chap who had been to Rampton. I had been told that Rampton was similar to Broadmoor except that a percentage of patients at Rampton were subnormal. The chap from Rampton had been locked up for seventeen years before being released. Broadmoor seemed shrouded in secrecy. It was as if people didn't really want to know or that they were frightened of knowing. I could only take in the few conflicting reports, mostly bad, that I had heard about it and the rest was left to the imagination. I was now considered a freak, a monster, with a dangerously uncertain future. It was difficult not to be despondent and the tears that day flowed quite naturally.

Twenty eight days after my trial I left Cardiff Jail hospital wing for the last time. I was leaving the scene of my greatest nightmare. I was pleased to be going but dreaded what awaited me.

I was however calm as I was processed at the reception area. After a few minutes everything was in order for me to leave for Berkshire. A car was waiting outside.

I was made to sit handcuffed between two prison officers I noted that there prime interest was the staff canteen at Broadmoor. I was just an incidental part of their day. The conversation reflected how much they had distanced themselves emotionally from the plight of those in their care and how they all too soon came to think of their charges as subhuman. Once on the journey one prison officer said:

"You'll do life."

I kept a brave face. I wasn't going to add to the amusement of the prison officers by a show of emotion. Anyway the countryside passing by me somehow helped my state of mind and there seemed no point in reacting anymore. Sometime later the prison officer said:

"Don't worry. You'll probably be out on the streets in eighteen months."

I felt a little relieved by that last remark. But the prison officer had not read Dr. Tidmarsh's report. I feared if he had he would not be so optimistic. After that conversation ran out. An hour later the car reached a crossroads and a little beyond that I noticed a sign:

"Broadmoor Special Hospital."

So I found myself in Broadmoor never having dreamt I would end up in such a place.

CHAPTER 12
BROADMOOR.

I hardly noticed the gatehouse to Broadmoor but inside I was vaguely conscious of a maze of redbrick buildings through which I was driven on my way to the admissions unit. Once out of the taxi a nurse ordered that my handcuffs be removed. The boot of the taxi was opened and another nurse took possession of my holdall. I then entered, the nurse following behind with my holdall in hand. I was pleasantly surprised on my admittance to discover an interior painted a light green. The improvement in the decor was some consolation for the grimness of my fate. The nurses were all dressed in the same outfit as the prison officers, they in fact belonged to the prison officers union but this was disguised by their wearing white medical coats.

Shortly after my arrival I was led to the bathroom by two nurses and I was made to step into a bath of lukewarm water, the traditional prison bath. After I had climbed out I was examined for any possible injuries and then a nurse said:

"You are in Broadmoor now. We don't stand for any nonsense. So watch it."

I had already decided to be as good as gold and as I had not laid a finger on anyone in Cardiff Jail I felt the warning unnecessary. But it was the only warning I was to receive and after it had been made I was given some pyjamas to put on and led to a side-room, really a cell with a bed in it. Standing at the open door a nurse told me that the window, a small slit looking onto the exercise yard, was of unbreakable glass. I was told to get off my bed if I heard a knock at the door. The door was then locked.

Periodically I noticed that I was being observed through the observation window next to the door. I listened closely for that knock but never did hear it suggesting that despite an exterior calm I was very troubled inside. An hour later a plate of food was placed inside the door. Accompanying it was a bowl of semolina. It was far superior to anything I had been given in prison and I ate it with relish.

A little later a junior doctor saw me in my side-room. I thought of him as my first means of escape. To escape I had to tell the truth I thought. So telling the truth was something I set about doing. I thought the best means of doing this was to repeat the saga of the nose. This I attempted to do.

After the meeting with the doctor I was given a dressing gown and slippers to put on and I was taken into the corridor. The charge nurse gave me a cigarette.

"The average stay here is four years ten months. When a person leaves he must be completely free of bitterness or resentment."

I took an instant liking to the charge nurse who was out to reassure me and just under five years did not seem an unendurably long time to be locked away for even though I thought I would do much longer than that and because of the nature of the psychiatric reports I looked at things in a pessimistic light.

"Tomorrow you can come out on association" he said.

I was again locked in my side-room.

The following morning, after the much needed respite of a night's sleep, I was shown to the washroom where I had to wait in a queue to shave. When my turn came and I had removed my top the nurses started at me:

"I don't like the sight of that right profile. The nose is rather bulbous."

I did not let their words bother me. I had far more serious things on my mind and as I had not been roused to anger by people mocking me about my appearance was not going to react now, particularly as the nurses clearly wanted a violent reaction. It was apparent to me that it had been accepted that my problem sprung from doubts about my self-image.

Back in my side-room I folded my blankets with the utmost meticulousness and placed them in a neat pile at the end of my bed. By being neat and tidy I hoped I might be able to get out of Broadmoor quicker though deep down I believed that nothing could prevent me from doing decades in Broadmoor. When a nurse came and noted my side-room all he said was:

"You have obviously been well trained in prison."

At ten o'clock I was allowed out on association. The dayroom was pleasantly decorated and wall-papered and all the chairs faced in one direction towards a coloured television set. I was surprised by the comfort. Ironically I was taken aback by how normal the other patients appeared. No one cried or shouted or was violent. I had hoped that I would stand out as normal from the rest and that would ensure a quicker discharge. But by behaving normally I realised that I would just blend in.

After five minutes I found I could not stand the thought of being a life prisoner any more even in this comparative luxury and I started to cry. A nurse came over and asked me why I was crying. I knew that it would achieve nothing by giving the real reason for my tears so I said:

"I was upset by the way I was teased over my nose this morning." I intended by that remark to continue the argument that I hoped would lead to my discharge from Broadmoor and the nurse

163

went and called the principle nurse responsible and he started to comfort me. That at least was a change from prison.

Even when my tears had dried and the nurse had gone I still felt wretched. "Stone walls do not a prison make." That line by Richard Lovelace was so simplistic now. Lovelace's prison only enclosed the body. His prisoner was blessed with hope of release. The walls of my prison enclosed not only my body but my mind. I was condemned to the bondage of zoo animals though zoo animals were at least able to mate and I wasn't. Even if the 1959 Mental Health Act had changed many things including how long a lunatic might spend in hospital it didn't seem that it could save me.

I tried to stop the brooding by having two or three games of snooker with another patient on a miniature snooker table in the dayroom. Having never played a proper game before I had to be told the rules. I then sat down in my chair again and tried to concentrate on the television which had been switched on so as to distract myself that way. All these activities did little to take my mind off the terrifying thought that I was here for good.

I looked around the dayroom noting all the patients and came to the conclusion that whatever anyone might have said about me in the past I was not homosexual but that if I was to survive I would have to turn myself that way. At that moment I felt incapable of responding sexually to any of the men in the room but homosexuality was something I would have to think about.

A black nurse interrupted my brooding when he took me to the medical room for a blood sample. He had a good bedside manner and at first I thought he was a doctor. He was very sympathetic and I thought: "They're not all bad."

Next I had to see the medical superintendent in an interview room in the ward. He was near retirement age and had a gentle manner but appreciating his awesome power I was rather nervous. My nervousness was probably justified for when one patient asked him seventeen years previously how long he would do, the same doctor had replied: "Seven times seven years". The patient had swung a punch, had been dragged to the refractory block and had his front teeth knocked out. He had taken the nurses to court and won and as a result was still serving a life stretch. The doctor went through Dr. Tidmarsh's report and asked: "Do you hear voices?" as if he thought I was badly out of touch with reality? I was sensible enough not to try and sway his ideas.

The chaplain in his black cassock paid me a visit easing himself down in an armchair next to me." I heard that you had a moral breakdown in prison" he said. What did he mean? Certainly my morale had been destroyed in prison.

After he had left I began to talk to another patient. He had drugged his two little girls then drowned then in the bath when his marriage began to break up. After that he took paraquat but recovered in hospital. He said it was to stop his children being sent to a home but that the doctors made out it was must revenge against his wife who had been committing adultery. Although I had heard of similar cases and the defendants had been freed doctors usually interpreted crimes in the worst way. Whether you reacted on remand in prison or not you could just as easily end up in a secure hospital. The patient, unlike me, had decided to show no emotion in prison.

As I talked to him I ascertained that he knew something about psychiatry. I said to him: "The doctors keep on asking me if I hear voices? I don't but should I say I do?"

"Not unless you want to do longer" he replied. I had found my only sensible piece of advice from a patient and after that he and I became close friends.

I met a friend of his who had a passion for drawing with pastels. His subject was an old farmhouse and he did several copies of the same scene which I thought were all perfect. He explained that the chiaroscuro was all wrong. He was in Broadmoor for causing £200 worth of criminal damage and said he had "cracked up" on remand. The reason for his crime was that he had been unemployed for seven years. Being sent to Broadmoor did seem a harsh punishment for such a minor offence. There appeared no set rhyme or reason for sending people to Broadmoor.

On the good side, at lunchtime I was allowed to eat in the dining room adjacent to the dayroom where I could have as much to eat as I wanted. The food had been transported by trolley from the kitchens behind the Central Hall and there was waiter service by other patients. I was able to eat with steel knives and forks as opposed to a plastic spoon in prison and the perpetual hunger that I had experienced in prison was finally abated.

That afternoon my parents visited. The visit was to last for two hours as opposed to the quarter of an hour I had been allowed in prison. As I didn't have any day clothes I saw them in an interview room on the ward rather than the Central Hall where visits normally took place. A waiter was summoned and I ordered coffee and biscuits. It was a very pleasant change to what I was used to in prison. The whole atmosphere contributed to a visible change in me which my parents noticed and the supervising nurse sat outside the interview room perfectly happy to let my parents and I discuss what we wanted. Halfway through the visit my father went and had a word with the nurse who was only too happy to be of assistance. After a relaxing two hours my parents were escorted out of the ward and I was shown back to the dayroom by the nurse. Just before we entered the dayroom he turned to me and said:

"Your parents love you very deeply. They both badly want you back. You haven't actually killed. You keep your nose clean and you will be out of here in no time." He mentioned the two patients I had spoken to that morning. "Don't hang around with them" he said. "They don't need you. You look after yourself."

I was very touched and grateful that he had shown such concern. However I doubted he had read Dr. Tidmarsh's report which was not encouraging and still weighed on me.

The next day I received my clothes for which I had been haphazardly measured the day before. They were all civvies and consisted of three shirts, a pair of pyjamas, two pairs of jeans and a brown striped suit. The suit which I tried on in front of the wall mirror in the gallery was so badly fitting that had not all other patients been similarly clad I would have been ashamed to wear it.

My room was changed to one in the main sleeping area of the ward. The ward was L shaped and my side-room was off the long stroke of the L. Before I went to bed I had to strip, fold, then hang up all my clothes in the locker on the wall of the gallery and walk naked to my side-room on the other side. There I put on my pyjamas which had been placed separately in my room. All this was supervised by nurses. I wondered with such a fool proof system how anyone could smuggle in an implement, rope or even tablets into his room if he wanted to do away with himself. My doubts over whether I had a future had reasserted themselves at this time and suicide seemed the only way out. The ultimate horror was that there was no possibility of committing suicide and so escaping the nightmare.

At nine o'clock the side-rooms were locked up. This was a very noisy business with four nurses walking abreast down the gallery, the one on the inside banging shut the doors of the side-rooms and locking them. The combined sound was like that of a train in motion.

That evening after locking up I examined my new side-room. Through the large barred window I could see a twenty feet high brick wall, the same wall that enclosed the whole hospital. I was separated from it by forty feet of grass and as it was night the wall was lit up by a search light. I had two large shutters in the inside of my window which I could open and close.

When silence fell finally upon the gallery I started to brood. As I was no longer on medication and as the largactil had had a strong tranquillising effect, something my body had learnt to combat, I was unable to sleep. It could take four years to get over the sense of desolation so I later established from one longstay patient and the beginning had to be the worst. For me there was no escape from my thoughts, again I felt trapped and in a state of nervous breakdown I started to blunder about my cell hammering against the walls with my fists. I then threw myself onto the bed covering my head with my pillow. But when the night nurse came by I pretended to be quite calm. On his return journey up the gallery I stopped him and explained that because I had been taken off drugs I was unable to sleep. He said he would mention my sleeplessness to the day staff in the morning.

The next morning nothing was said about my sleeplessness the previous night but I had other things to occupy my mind for after breakfast there was ward work. As I had not had any day clothes before and as my holdall had been sent to the stores containing what clothes I had I had been exempt from this. Now I was told to clean out the toilets and I did this with pride and meticulousness. I was out to create a good impression. Everything I did was calculated to getting out of Broadmoor even if I believed I was hoping against hope.

On the Saturday I went down to the football field at the bottom of the terrace in front of the hospital; and from there I was able to ascertain the general layout of the hospital. The male section was E shaped and consisted of seven houses, Gloucester, Kent, Dorset, Somerset, Essex (a less secure block for "parole" patients), Norfolk (the refractory block), and Cornwall. The middle stroke of the E consisted of the Central Hall on the ground floor and the chapel above. There was also a school. On the right were the two female houses, Lancaster and York.

At the football field I started to wander amongst the patients listening carefully to what people had to say. I gathered that many people like me looked upon Broadmoor as a psychiatric prison and that it had formerly been called a Criminal Lunatic Asylum. It reputedly housed some of the most dangerous men and women in Britain, some with crimes not only serious but eccentric. One patient was said to have cut off his victim's head and cooked it in an oven. But many patients were perfectly harmless.

A few days later I started in the assessment unit. This was situated in a lean-to and it was through going there that I made my first acquaintance with Mr Sharp. It was his job to escort patients from my house, Somerset house, to the lean-to where he would supervise them. He had worked in Broadmoor in the days before the 1959 Mental Health Act when patients rarely got out. While I was in the assessment unit I was more interested in him than doing carpentry or handicrafts for I hoped he might have some consoling words to offer. He was an interesting fund of information saying for example that a chap who had been sent to prison for the term of his natural life had then been transferred to Broadmoor where he had only done seven years. But he did not say anything hopeful to me except that "the wheels of Broadmoor grind very slowly." There was a patient working alongside me whom I took more seriously. He had been locked up for thirteen years for a comparatively minor offence and his story filled me with horror.

A week or two after my arrival at Broadmoor I received a visit from an acquaintance called Ray Bevan. I was now receiving visits in the Central Hall which was also used for conferences, film shows and dances. It also had a stage for theatricals. The business going there had been fairly complex for as with all patient movements there was locking and unlocking, head counting and monitoring by radio. At our table I ordered a pot of coffee and a packet of biscuits from the canteen next door. The canteen was really a shop selling most of what you could wish for in the way of eats and soft drinks and the patients went to the canteen once a week to stock up on food and cigarettes. I paid for the coffee out of my weekly allowance.

Although having a visit was always a pleasant occasion this time there was a set purpose for it for Ray, having heard from my uncle and aunt in the Orange Free State where he had worked, that I was in Broadmoor, hoped he might be able to offer me a way out through religion. He had been told by the chaplain that I would do very many years in Broadmoor. We talked at length on the subject of religion but it soon became apparent that though I would have dearly liked any way out I could not rekindle any spark of my former faith. The conversation turned to other matters. But Ray thereafter gave me continuous support even though he remained mystified by the fact that people who had murdered had been let off whilst I who hadn't was doing life.

About two weeks after my arrival in Broadmoor I decided to write down on paper a brief summary of my case for the doctors. It started off on a modest scale but was eventually extended to cover fifteen pages of foolscap. Unfortunately I was terrified of disagreeing with the doctors who had the power to throw away the key on me so I kept on using words like "mission", "punishment", "paranoid", "attack", words that had been used by the doctors to describe what happened before. I also over emphasised any feelings of hostility towards Enid. But I had this feeling that what had been said could not be unsaid and I simply wanted to knock on the head any suggestion of paranoid schizophrenia.

After three weeks I was asked to pack all my belongings in a black bin liner and I was escorted upstairs to the middle ward, the adolescent unit. It was for under twenty fives and I gathered its purpose was to try and prevent the younger patients being contaminated by the older ones. On my arrival I was shown round the ward by a nurse then left to acquaint myself with the other patients. There were about twenty five in all. There was also much less supervision than in the admissions unit. I missed the cocooned feeling of the downstairs ward but assumed that to have moved so quickly to this less stringent regime might suggest that the staff had some trust in me; as trust was the principal factor in a patient's discharge I hoped that I was now nearer the gate.

The ward was fairly commodious. There were bars on the windows but otherwise there was all the space you could require and I was permitted to wander between the dayroom, the scullery and the dining room. In the dayroom there were the facilities that there had been downstairs and I could make tea or coffee in the scullery during free time.

I got talking to a patient called Tony seated in two armchairs in an alcove in the dayroom. Tony was black-haired and Italianate. We got onto talking about our case histories. I myself, as usual, was more interested in gleaning information than in imparting it. Tony had stabbed a woman during an attempted burglary and had been locked up for four years. I wondered if the doctors considered him homicidal. I also wondered if I would be sitting in the same armchair in four years time. Somehow it still seemed that I would only leave the hospital in a "wooden box" and what Tony had to say did nothing to dispel that fear.

Three or four days later I had my first interview with Dr. U.. He was the doctor responsible for adolescent patients. He was one of seven consultant psychiatrists in Broadmoor and was termed a god. As said I had already appreciated Dr. P. was to all intents and purposes a god. Your future as a patient in Broadmoor depended on your consultant psychiatrist who was not only omnipotent but believed himself omniscient. I was soon to find out that as with most psychiatrists, once a Broadmoor psychiatrist had made up his mind about you, nothing in the world would change it. It was his opinion that mattered. Even the chair the doctor sat in was termed the god chair. So that lunchtime I sat in the charge nurse's office before Dr. U., the Most High. Three other nurses were also present in the room and with me I had my summary.

I proceeded with my case. I was used to being allowed one minute or less in which to say what I wanted for that was all the time Dr. P. permitted me in prison and so I tried to get everything out within that time limit. Dr. U. took in not the words but the manner of delivery and after I had finished he simply said:

"You're mad, potty, round the bend, off your rocker, crazy, barmy, loony" or words to that effect. He had taken my rapidity of speech as a manic sign and though I had made it obvious that I had been worried about my nose because I did not look like a Frankenstein monster my preoccupation was misread to signify that I was deluded about my looks. He I discovered described me as labile which I was not. He said:

"You don't feel any remorse." He must have read Dr. Tidmarsh's report and must therefore have assumed I was not only schizophrenic but guilty of all the worst charges levelled at me. I still felt that I had not done anything more than make a scene and certainly my deep down intentions had not gone beyond that. A display of remorse would thus have been illogical though I obviously regretted the consequences to myself. Had I injured Enid I know I would have felt terrible but the only one hurt was me. So keeping tight-lipped I pulled out my summary and left it on the desk in the office. Dr. U. didn't even glance at it. I felt I had done all I could to try and sort out the mess that I was in.

That evening after the four o'clock teas I was instructed to wait in the medicine queue and when my turn came was given haloperidol. A nurse who had been present in the charge nurse's office that lunchtime and who was supervising the queue said:

"Write to MIND, consult your MP, refer the matter to the Court of Human Rights in Strasbourg, you are now on drugs."

For better or for worse I was now back on drugs even though I was beginning to adapt to being off them and in addition to the return of my hyperventilation, all the other awful side effects were to resume.

That night I thought about my dilemma. No one was interested in my side of the story. Ever since my arrival at Cardiff Jail a chain reaction had set in where, with a few reservations, what Dr. P. had said was immediately echoed in some form by subsequent psychiatrists. A dominant personality always had his view accepted and though Dr. U. was reputed to be fair, intelligent, wise and well-intentioned where patients were concerned I saw it would be impossible to sway the main body of opinion. I had gathered that one stage to discharge involved admitting, guilty or innocent, to your alleged offence. A nurse went on to say that but for the" grace of god" I would be a murderer. In fact it was the reverse, but for the very worst bad luck ever known I would be happy and free with no criminal record. But because the medical staff had this false picture of me I would have to admit to that. At that stage I was not ready to sell my soul but decided to at least display some contrition though I had hurt no one for as the doctors were not treating me, but a fiction, I would have to imagine myself as that fiction and respond like it. I would play along with the doctors. At the same time I would do so in a way that might benefit me rather than hurting me too much. I was on drugs and drugs were obviously given for a purpose, in this case treat schizophrenia though my whole notion of such a thing was to radically alter once I saw through the label. Thus I decided I would pretend to be a so-called schizophrenic and I would stage a dramatic recovery. It was a gamble but with so many misconceptions about me I had nothing to lose by play-acting.

The next day I said to the nurses I was feeling much better, that my self-confidence had improved immeasurably and that I no longer saw anything wrong with my nose. In fact I was always able to see the imperfections and how I fell short of perfection though in some lights I could see why some might say it was okay. I had to say it was all right to suggest I was all right. As they felt the drugs were necessary to bring about such a change in viewpoint I took them up on this. In point of fact my mental machinery already retarded through depression now had to endure the effects of the "liquid cosh". On top of this being looked upon as a complete lunatic can only be bad for a person's self-confidence.

A few days later I again saw Dr. U. in the charge nurse's office.

"You have made a remarkable recovery" he said. "You have suffered an acute illness. You are now convalescing."

My act had been successful, but I could not help feeling just a little guilt that Dr. U., one of the few psychiatrists I had met who at that stage I liked should have to think such a thing though I had gone a long way to recovery anyway and it was just my indefinite incarceration that made me anxious and terribly depressed. If I had not tended always to look for the good in people I would have seen that there had not been any real effort to understand me and that I had just been summarily made out to be mad.

Shortly after that I became the victim of a prank by three of my fellow patients. One of the patients had been a skinhead who I was told killed for pleasure. Another had raped and assaulted an old lady who had died inhaling her own blood. The third was physically very strong and possessed a deadly fist but was not as bad as the other two. However all three had taken an instantaneous dislike to me because I was gentle and subdued though they had concealed the fact up till then. All I knew was that my name was being called over the tannoy when I was summoned to the office. There I was presented with a pair of grossly soiled underpants.

"Are these yours?" asked a nurse.

I had a look at the underpants and then at the name tag on which my number was also marked. As the name and the number were mine I could not very well deny that the underpants were mine as well. But I did deny that I was responsible for the mess inside them. Obviously they had been dirtied deliberately to try and discredit me in the eyes of the staff and patients. It did not appear like human excrement that was used but mud from the playing field and I was believed when I said I had nothing to do with the soiling of the underpants. They were sent to the laundry and came back in tatters they were put through the washing machine so many times.

After that I was careful with whom I associated. The three aforementioned patients were not to be looked upon as ideal living companions for me. And such people had a label – psychopaths. If there were exceptions to the rule such people were usually aloof, difficult get on with, fastidious, aggressive immoral, brutish and insensitive. They regarded inadequacy as the ultimate evil and were largely evil.

However I now appreciated that for someone in my position, to start bandying about the word evil would be dangerous. Evil was a word I rarely heard used in Broadmoor and in describing destructive or immoral behaviour the word used was psychopathic, not evil as someone brought up with a Christian background like mine might say. But it appeared to go even deeper than this and I was beginning to learn that the hospital's philosophy was run on Darwinist rather than Christian lines. I would have expected there to be an emphasis on reforming patients but the reality was that there was little or no talk of what was moral or immoral as such, only what was legal or illegal. To me that meant that people with power or influence amongst patients and staff were given carte blanche to practise psychological abuse and that as with the case of Enid, the law was liable to become a weapon rather than a safeguard. I was thus to refer to Enid's behaviour as psychopathic rather than evil. My view on things had and could not change, only my terminology.

I transferred all my attentions to the other patients. These were largely "schizophrenic" though there was a smattering of normals, neurotics and depressives amongst them. The schizophrenics who bordered on being inadequate at least in the Broadmoor environment, rather than deluded or out of touch with reality, had the appellation "goons" and formed the lowest stratum of hospital society. However amongst them there was always someone to talk to. One patient who was normal most of the time and neurotic part of the time was even sympathetic towards me saying I should never have been sent to Broadmoor, a view he consistently held. He had been raped and held at chisel-point for twenty four hours in the hospital. His attacker and an accomplice later took another patient hostage, buggering him, then cutting off his genitals. The torture lasted four hours before their victim pleaded with them to put him out of his misery when they strangled him with cheese wire. The motive was to return to prison. The first patient was interestingly middle class and I had a lot of time for him. It was noteworthy how I tended to get on better with middle class patients than with working class ones whose poor backgrounds had often been responsible for a bad set of morals and a law of the jungle philosophy.

On the whole though the patients did not care for me or my predicament. So insecure were they over their own situations that they frequently delighted in the misfortunes of others. I found that few patient wanted to listen to my tale of woe and were hostile to me when I broached the subject. I was on my own and very

172

much alone. But when it came down to it it was not the patients that worried me, only the question of how long I would do. The patients were merely representative of the more brutish elements outside and I resolved never to let a patient get the better of me or to drive me to violence.

I found my name had been put down for a disco and not having had any congenial female company for five months I decided to go. I hoped that being able to associate with women for a couple of hours once a month might ease the pain of such an unnatural existence. So one evening I was escorted along with about twenty others from Somerset house to the top ward in York house. The discotheque in York house was small and compact but was very agreeable in comparison to the rest of the female wing. It had been fitted through the fund-raising activities of Jimmy Savile, a frequent visitor to the hospital and the only outsider with the keys to Broadmoor. But though the disco had a welcoming feeling the sight of the women was not so warming. Someone from outside taken along to a disco was told: "Now every woman in here has killed someone." That might not have been accurate or fair. But certainly in terms of looks they were the most prepossessing bunch of women I had met. I did notice a couple of attractive female nurses but it was a sin for a patient to fancy a nurse. I couldn't however be choosy about women anymore and the women, who were outnumbered seven to one by the men in the hospital soon became very choosy about the men they associated with. Although some patients objected to the way their dealings with the women patients were monitored and recorded I hoped I might be able to get discos to work for me.

I had seated myself at an empty table together with Tony. There were tables and chairs all round the edge of the disco and on the tables were bowls of crisps and peanuts. There were soft drinks at the door. Tony and I helped ourselves to the peanuts. After about ten minutes the disco had filled to capacity with the gradual entrance of more female patients. The music was pounding and a few patients were twisting and jiving on the dance floor. I felt it about time I joined them and after I had plucked up sufficient courage I wandered over to a female patient and asked her for a dance. Fortunately she agreed but after the record was over I said thank you and promptly sat down again before she could walk away. Despite having had one dance I felt very nervous and desolate as I sat amongst all those unprepossessing women. I had hoped that as such they might at least show a little bit of interest in me. I was ignored. My confidence, already at a low ebb ran even lower. I was however grateful to be amongst women.

Towards the end of the disco I livened up and had a few more dances. Tony just sat at our able watching, and although one haggard old woman who possessed the regrettable delusion that the food was poisoned never refused me a dance, I did wonder how women rated me now. When I was escorted back to the ward afterwards I felt a mixture of relief at having experienced some female company but down-hearted by their reaction to me.

At around this time I received a visit from Jerome. We sat in the visiting hall with a pot of coffee in front of us. He had been asked to visit by my mother who together with my father had paid me regular visits from Devon and who didn't want me just to rot in captivity. Jerome in the true spirit of friendship had responded to her request though not understanding the nature of a life sentence thought me self-preoccupied. He again came up with a school friend who was at medical school. Despite his visit I did feel very isolated from the outside world. More than that I now hoped that the outside world might rescue me from my prison. Only Tony, Nick and perhaps a couple of others at university could secure my freedom by amplifying certain statements made and by supplying new information and so revealing the whole truth. I decided to write to them and get them to visit. I also wrote to my two old English masters and my old Biology master at school. I was anxious for some worthwhile contact and my middle-aged English master had brought out the best in me at school. I did not forget Mr Griffiths , my only legal advisor to make any real attempt to defend me. I wrote a courtesy letter to the Cardiff solicitors and finally I wrote to Julie.

A few days later I received a reply to my letter to Tony. He wrote: "It is the person who treats a rational person irresponsibly who is the guilty party." It was the first time that anyone had acknowledged that Enid's cruel psychological games were at least irresponsible. He said that they all thought I was going to get a sentence totally out of proportion to the "little thing" I did. He promised to visit and bring up some friends with him in his car.

I then received a reply to my letter to Julie. She thought it an act of gross injustice that I should have been sent to Broadmoor and wrote: "Il non carborundum illegitimi." She said that the president of the students union at Lampeter had passed the news around that I had been sent to Broadmoor and that a doctor had labelled me schizophrenic and she was anxious for me to put the blame for all that had happened on my friends teasing me in public over my nose and for me to be freed on appeal. She even suggested that I write to the Court of Human Rights in Strasbourg or the Commission of Civil Liberties not knowing that outside courts and civil bodies could not and never would succeed in influencing the might of the doctors and the Home Office.

My two old English masters were also very prompt to reply and promised to visit. It was pleasant to know that at least a couple of people had retained a modicum of respect for me.

In Mr Griffiths reply to my letter he was very flattering saying that I had a lot to offer "the community at large." He was keen to help and felt that I could use my time in Broadmoor studying for a degree with the Open University, though he would not have known that I was too depressed to concentrate on study and that because of the drugs I could not sit still enough to read a book properly.

Eventually I received a reply to my letter to Nick who also promised to visit but with the exception of saying how shocked he was at my condition in jail and asking me to be best man at his wedding to Lorna I saw that his words were, like those of most charming people, empty.

And when I wrote back to Julie rejecting her theory that my friends teasing me in public had been the trigger she cut me off. Except for one more letter from Nick I was to hear no more from my friends after that.

Though I had been abandoned by most of the young generation I still had the older generation and one weekend I received a visit from a couple called the Simpsons whom I had briefly met when I was younger. They were long standing friends of my parents and lived in Gerrards Cross. As they were relatively close to Broadmoor they had volunteered to visit me and proved to be exceptionally kind, generous and understanding. We were seated at one of the tables in the visiting hall. Mrs Simpson remarked: "I can't see any murderers." I chirped back: "They're all around you." She couldn't believe that murderers could appear so normal, but though I enjoyed their visit I really wanted the sort of visit that would bring me help. No one did come with the help that I required.

I soon saw that the outside world was a dead loss. There were my parents who had now incidentally started upon a move to Hampshire to be near me. There were the Simpsons and a couple of other friends of my parents who were a continuous support. But when it came down to actual positive help I saw that I had been thoroughly let down by the outside. All that was left for me to do was to construct a life inside.

Inside there were a few patients who offered warmth and friendship. One young lad I liked a lot. He had caused a few pounds worth of arson and by a twist in his fortunes had ended up in Moss Side. Arsonists were viewed with tremendous suspicion by the doctors. The argument was that if you dropped a lighted cigarette on the floor it could set alight to the carpet, burn down the room, spread through the building and engulf a street. This argument I disapproved of. In Moss Side the patient had bided his time and more than once was told he was leaving when he wasn't. He lost faith with the representatives of authority. It was felt Dr. U. could straighten him out and release him.

Another patient I liked was David Winter. He was a very good technical artist painting in meticulous detail creatures of the wild in particular birds of prey. He had been expelled from public school for poaching. He used to snare rabbit and catch pheasant for the boys. One day the boys said: "Oh, come on Dave. How about mutton for a change?" In a stupid dare he ventured out with an axe. Things turned into a bit of a nightmare with the axe bouncing off the sheep's head causing it to bolt and with Dave blundering about in tears in the semi-darkness with the thought of putting it out of its misery. He also sent a live frog and later a cat's tail through the post to a woman. People might have said: "Poor woman." I commented: "My sympathy lay with the frog." In consequence he was remanded in custody. He had a macabre fascination for Broadmoor and had wanted to come.

Another chap I liked had been given a five year sentence in prison but at the end had been transferred to Broadmoor. He burned down a school causing £5,000,000 worth of damage.

I also liked John Neish and spent an afternoon walking round the football pitch with him. He had punched an old lady and had been remanded in custody. It was a tremendous shock to be told that she had died of complications. He received eight years and ended up in Parkhurst. He complained how he was unable to face a sentence that long, he had been interviewed by a Broadmoor doctor and went to Broadmoor to complete his sentence. He was a good poet, he later read some of it on television. He spoke of his need for an "anchor", his seascape verse extended the idea and he proved an interesting companion.

Despite my few cronies in my heart I still felt desolated. I continued to live with the dream of being free again, of being able to go down to the pub for a drink, of being able to have girlfriends, even of one day getting married, of being a normal person doing all the things that make up a normal life. But that was impossible in Broadmoor. It was like an island cut off from the rest of society. Inside there were still barriers to break down and I felt a bit like Robinson Crusoe. I could not escape the fact that I was just a number without rights, state-owned forever.

I started working out how long I would do asking patients about themselves and their offenses. One patient who had committed petty larceny had been locked up for eight years. His story was not uncommon and it made me wonder how long someone who faced the serious charges I had to face would do.

There was a chap on my ward who had been transferred from prison after seven years for shooting his girlfriend in a supermarket. In prison he could have expected to do ten years, three years for manslaughter. But for murder or manslaughter you could expect to do seventeen to twenty five years in a special hospital. He was not even halfway through his "sentence". It was almost better in the eyes of the law to be bad than mad (though things have changed a lot since then.)

There were many cases of people who were far more suited to a semi-secure environment than a top security hospital and even where counsel or treatment might have helped , an institution such as Grendon Underwood would have been far better permitting a fixed sentence and thus parity in terms of years and months served. There was one such case of a chap who had been convicted of attempted rape, he had been on the ward for seven years and had suffered through being sent to Broadmoor.

A chap called Peter Utting, a policeman's son, was too clever for his own good and when asked why he did what he did by a Broadmoor doctor replied: "A little green worm in my head told me to do it." That guaranteed he was sent to Broadmoor and had done five years for a comparatively minor offence. In his case Broadmoor had just been treated as a dumping ground.

There were also cases of people in Broadmoor who were supposed to be a danger to themselves. As it was not a criminal offence to commit suicide and as I felt it was everyone's right to kill himself should the pressure become unbearable I was a little dismayed at that discovery.

My occupational therapist said I would do twelve years. I estimated that I would do from twelve years to natural life. The thought was depressing beyond measure.

Even now I was considering the possibility of an appeal. A young, friendly, female solicitor called Miss King came to see me on the ward. We were given the interview room to talk in. As I sat down I accidentally leaned against the alarm button causing a rush of nurses to the room. Miss King was not ruffled and seeing that I had not attacked her and she was all right they left. Miss King told me that she had read the report made at "Carmarthen General Hospital" but that she had not seen the other reports yet so an assessment of my chances at an appeal had not been made. Again devastating reports drawing on evidence fabricated in statements to the police were being used for an assessment. At this stage Miss King did seem quite optimistic and offered to come down on the train to see me again. I was dubious and told her not to bother. Only two percent of people who applied for tribunals were freed and they had done next to nothing. I had given up hope of an appeal.

One day in the assessment unit, after having been told by my parents that a girl I knew from my pre-school days in South Africa was getting married, I had a daydream about returning to the

177

great and bustling city of Durban. I thought of Durban's long sandy beaches, of the rickshaw boys gaily whisking their fares along the promenade, of the high skyscrapers rising up behind. But the reality of that little shed in which I did my joints and made my unsatisfactory baskets, the fact that I was in Broadmoor and that Broadmoor was my home and that it might as well have been the whole universe, made that dream ever more painful.

Later I was told I was to be moved to the workshops. They were an alternative to the handicrafts and consisted of the tailors, the leather shop, the printers, the television workshops, the Chronicle office where the patients magazine was printed, and the carpenters. I had written in a letter to my parents that I was interested in the printers and so I was given a job in the bookbinders which was part of the printers. All letters were censored and the fact that this little detail had been noted showed how carefully letters were vetted.

When I arrived there the first thing that I noticed was how many knives there were about. As two patients I was with in the assessment unit had stabbed to death people outside I was moved to take note of the knives. There were many other sharp implements that also took my notice but the thought of the danger did not affect me. I just thought that I must be regarded with some trust to have been placed amongst all these dangerous weapons.

The bookbinders proved preferable to the assessment unit. It also offered me a new trade and a fellow bookbinder got me to fold some blank sheets into booklets. These I had to sew together and glue. I then cut out two boards for a back and front cover on the guillotine. With some scissors I cut out some plastic, a spine and two fly leaves. I pasted on the plastic on the boards and then the spine, folded the edges and fitted the cover on my book. I was to create several albums like this. Indeed having developed a love of books and literature I liked the idea of being a bookbinder and had a chance to read certain of the journals and books on medicine which I had to bind for the medical library. I found out little about psychiatry that I did not already know but over time read the disturbing accounts of a couple of patients I knew who had been mentioned in books on psychiatry.

Most importantly I was happy with my occupational therapist, who not only understood printing but who was a stabilising influence on the patients. He proved to be of immeasurable worth for I needed someone around who was both reliable, consistent and understanding.

But if my freedoms had been increased I remained concerned by how I could obtain my complete freedom, the only freedom that really mattered to me. As said, I was far from alone in this. Complete freedom was the dream of virtually every patient. Some actually thought of achieving it by getting over the wall. But even if you did get over the wall where could you go? The siren was tested every morning and you could expect the alarms to go off and the neighbouring countryside to be swarming with police and soldiers in a matter of minutes. You could guarantee you would be mentioned on the television and the radio. All patients had their photographs taken because of the possibility of escape. And who would harbour an escaped mental patient? A mother who attempted to help her son escape received a lengthy prison sentence.

So I pestered my occupational therapist and the nurses in the ward with all manner of questions designed deep down to find out how long I would do, especially if I would do longer than the ten years that I personally felt I could endure. Much heartache and discussion could have been saved by some convincing reassurance and I tended to look upon escape as a well nigh impossible task.

At this time the idea of my doing an Open University course was briefly mooted. Down at the games field I discussed the subject with Alan Reeve. My concentration was not up to it and as I still wondered if I had a future I wondered about the point of it. As Alan Reeve and I strolled together he said: "Well you know it's not a Mickey Mouse degree." In the hospital it was usually only those with psychopathic labels who took Open University degrees. They were more likely to stay the course whereas those with artistic temperaments, the more imaginative or creative were rarely considered for it.

Although rare stories of violence filtered back to me I saw little of it between staff and patients. Despite the occasional breach of discipline, discipline remained remarkably effective taking into account the reputedly low tolerance levels of many patients and the stresses and strains faced by them. The security was such that bad behaviour could only be counterproductive even if you imagined you were going to be locked up in perpetuity. Everything was designed to make you conform. The carrot to behave well was an increase in privileges such as a privileged room and for the majority of patients the chance of one day earning your freedom. The stick was the "bang up" room or seclusion, a loss of privileges such as going to the canteen or being sent to Norfolk house, the refractory block (intensive care). Though you could go to Norfolk house and still be offered the chance of a discharge I was careful avoid the possibility of being sent there or to seclusion which I saw as a few steps back from the gate. A small black chap was on the ward for three weeks, but he had a loud laugh that consistently rang through the ward and he was then carted off to Norfolk house.

At this time a male psychologist appeared o the ward. We sat down in the interview room and I had to do a I.Q. test for him. I was asked questions such as : "What is the meaning of blood is thicker than water?" I had to repeat numbers read out to me, the

179

numbers getting one digit longer each time. The truth was rather than do tests I would have preferred to discuss my problems, particularly that of being a patient without limit of time in Broadmoor. For me this was like being faced with a giant abyss and the consequent depression was so profound my memory was defective, I had been unable to remember anything from my French grammar which I had dipped into and my thought processes had slowed down to a snail's pace. Although I did score above average in the test it was not reflective of me at my best and anyway I remained highly sceptical over such tests which assessed less than twenty five out of ten thousand types of intelligence and the talented people at such tests I discovered were psychic which was a normal adult development. My values meant that I still tended to look up to a good artist or thinker and I measured people's abilities differently and far more reliably. By talking to the psychologist I had hoped to rectify the mistake that had led to my being sent to Broadmoor, gauge how long I might be likely to do and find the key to my getting out of Broadmoor. I was just left to endure the experience, the pain was as bad as I had known and with my nerves shattered by my life sentence I presented as inadequate. Before I walked out of the door I was handed a multiphasic personality test to complete.

My relationship with my social worker was more productive and I discussed details of my case with him in the interview room on the ward. His prime concern was to find out about my previous home life and with helping my parents with any difficulties relating to my being in Broadmoor. I mentioned a couple of things such as how my mother would get annoyed with my father when he went out in the car without informing her. The social worker was even to go all the way down to Devon to visit my parents gathering a favourable impression. I still enjoyed a close relationship with them. As I was anxious for an ear I regarded these interviews as important even though my deep-rooted fears that what had been written about me precluded a future, remained.

I was asked to see another psychologist and was escorted to the psychology department. He was doing a thesis for his Ph.D on the encephalograph and turned out to be very understanding and gentle. Although he had been sent the psychiatric reports on me beforehand he remained unaffected and regarded them with open scepticism. But his prime concern was to measure my reactions and give me an E.E.G.. He seated me in a hardbacked chair and gave me a handpiece with a button attached to a flex. I had to press the button in response to signals given to me. He wired a number of electrodes to my head and measured my brainwaves. The E.E.G. was able to show up immature brainwaves and otherwise abnormal brainwave patterns. I later discovered that my brainwave patterns were normal. I found the whole experience with the psychologist both salutary and informative though despite meeting the odd individual with a grasp of psychology I still felt that I had been shut away forever from a normal life and that these isolated people could not help me.

A few days before Christmas our ward had its Christmas party. This took place in a Nissen hut in the hospital grounds and a few specially selected females from York and Lancaster were invited. The male patients went over first and David and I chose a table. The Nissen hut was adorned with decorations and in a corner was a table full of eats and soft drinks. The female patients arrived and a slim, auburn-haired, bespectacled girl came and sat down opposite me. Though she was not pretty I still regarded such a thing as a great honour in my present circumstances. She asked me for a dance and we rose and walked onto the dance floor. She had a boyfriend in another house, a formidable sporting male though she made out he was too possessive. Amazingly there were a couple of pretty girls among the patients and they were being chatted up by a couple of the psychopathic killers including the skinhead turned killer. I was learning that a bully was the mark of a man and was leading me to alter my notion that men were only graded by women according to how good looking they were.

Though lacking the qualities to score a hit with the pretty girls I was able to enjoy the Christmas just a little. The ward had been covered with tinsel and decorations and boasted a fine Christmas tree with fairy lights. Having been given a few days off from the bookbinders the holiday was complete. However I did not attend chapel on Christmas day, not because many staff regarded the need for a faith as a mark of weakness but because I had simply become a confirmed atheist.

After Christmas the clinical question started again when I was invited downstairs for my case conference. There the superintendent said in front of everyone that I had nearly caused a "terrible tragedy". My view, though I did not express it, was that Enid was never in serious danger and that the tragedy was what happened to me, not Enid. As she was a force in the world, her well being was considered but mine not at all though I was the only one who had come close to death. In other ways I tried to be open with the result that the case conference proved inconclusive.

The next day I had to see Dr. U. in the charge nurse's office and he asked me if I thought I had been deluded adding that he and the nurses present thought I had been. Frightened to go out on a limb I said "yes" without believing it. That marked the end of my dealings with psychiatrists for sometime. It was decided I was now ready for group therapy.

Up till now I had been left to treat myself other than for the unwelcome fact of being put on drugs. I had assumed that it was the policy amongst nurses and doctors to let you ,the patient, work things out for yourself. But I still doubted that even to have done that was to have got much closer to the gate. A patient in another ward had been told that despite having made his recovery he would now have to do his punishment. But when I was told to stay on the ward for "group" instead of going to work one day, I hoped that on group the medical staff would at least be able to offer me the benefit of some of their expert knowledge. The group took place in the dayroom and comprised ten male patients from the upstairs ward and from my ward and a doctor who chaired the group. The members of the group all sat round in a circle in armchairs and one or two nurses joined in.

What first became apparent was that the more voluble ones on the group were also the more eccentric ones or the ones who were most unhappy about their confinement and I quickly learnt all I wanted to know about them. One had burned down his parents house. I had first met him a month or two previously when I went up to him and asked him how long he had done. He had replied: "Fuck off." The reason was that he was obsessed with getting out and this later led him to attempt suicide by cutting his wrists with the lid of a food tin. Another patient had stabbed his brother and described the stabbing on the group. He said the sensation was like stabbing a paper bag. He had " worked his passage" to Broadmoor because he had been wrongly told that he would do a shorter time in Broadmoor than in prison. He took the whole set up very lightly and described himself as a "latent heterosexual" which was his way of poking fun at the establishment which suspected all patients of being homosexual. He was a brilliant wit and once quipped: "The answer to Broadmoor is morphine." But his whole attitude had incurred the wrath of the doctors. A third patient was intensely religious and though he had only committed a minor offence and was on section 60 had been locked up for ten years. He was "pumped" with drugs and constantly maintained that all the drugs did for him was to make him "drunk". He had been raped by a group of patients in the hospital and because he had submitted was deemed an incurable homosexual. He had attempted to hang himself from his upturned bed causing all the blood vessels in his face to burst. A charge nurse told him that if he gave up religion he would get out. He thus went on to renounce his faith on the group. The group that first day left me more informed and more worried. But I was relieved to discover that though there was E.C.T., lobotomies
were not carried out in the hospital because of the risk of death.

But I couldn't exist purely on group therapy which usually avoided the most pressing issue anyway, that of my captivity. I couldn't exist purely on the stodgy diet of Broadmoor either. To exist in a meaningful sense I still needed warmth and a purpose.

It was at this stage that I attempted an affair with Tony. It was evening and he and I were sitting at a table in the dining room during a recreation period. Suddenly I felt his leg touch mine through my jeans. My first thought was to move my leg away. Something told me to let it remain. Gradually I felt the heat of his leg communicate itself to mine.

After about a minute or two and without a word from me, we rose from our chairs and surreptitiously made our way to the sleeping area of the ward. He stood close to me and stared into my eyes longingly. But seeing the short growth of stubble on his face I found I could not bring myself to kiss him and we decided to make our way back to the main part of the ward.

I might have failed in my last attempt to find a way out but things did improve when I was granted a privileged room. In my room I was allowed a television and a record player in addition to my bed, cupboard and desk. Instead of being confined during the day to the main part of the ward I could spend my time in my privileged room and I remember lying on my bed one day reading Lust for Life, the tragic novel of Van Gogh. It was one of several books I borrowed from the mobile library. Although I still felt trapped forever in some nightmare world my pain reaching to a depth many times greater than that at Lampeter University, my room provided a hideaway in which I could shelter from grim reality.

At some point a patient on the ward died and my numbed reaction to this illustrated just how much I was preoccupied with my own pain and horror at my "life sentence" at the time. I was walking down the gallery past the patient's side-room one morning when I glanced through the door which was standing ajar and inside I saw the patient sitting in a chair. He had complained of a headache the previous evening and now his head was swollen up like a pumpkin and he was staring blankly ahead of him as if he was totally unaware of what was going on round him. It was obvious by his ghastly condition that he wouldn't survive and on being taken to a general hospital soon died. There was a wave of sympathy generated through the hospital by the news, meningitis was suspected leading to talk of us all being inoculated and it was argued the patient should have been treated earlier. But as a patient upstairs commented: "What's everybody so worried about? He's out of it now." And rather than sorrow those were my sentiments.

That Holy Week two Franciscan brothers and a sister came on a mission to the hospital and on Good Friday they held a pageant in the chapel which I was moved to attend. One of the brothers staggered up the aisle bearing a giant cross, at the chancel steps a patient relieved him of his load and then two patients crucified him at the altar. Hanging from the cross in a convincing simulation of the passion he cried out: "Oh God, why hast thou forsaken me?" A common cry in Broadmoor. By Easter he had had his resurrection and preached a brilliant sermon in chapel which I was also moved to attend. The two brothers left the hospital having made a number of conversions. I still only put my faith in one so-called god, Dr. U.. He at least could work the miracle of a discharge and very soon the converts of the brothers lost their faith. They lost it when they lost their belief in a traditional god working miracles for them.

All the time new patients were being admitted onto the ward displacing some who had been on the ward for a long time and who were moved onto more senior wards. I found out a lot about the new patients from newspapers and on occasions the television which I saw as a useful source of information. Only Ronnie Kray, soft spoken and polite, who was in the upstairs ward, was famous. Others just enjoyed a brief blaze of notoriety. One had killed his mother and "guardian" with a pair of scissors when they lay in bed. He had been broken by his "life sentence" contributing to a look of inadequacy and had been told by a junior doctor that he would never get out. He like me, had a schizophrenic label, the fate of the subdued male, and was further reduced by drugs when if anyone it was a handful of the aggressive psychopaths who would have benefitted from drug suppression. A second patient had buggered a baby, he was just immature and had been transferred from Borstal to Broadmoor at the end of his sentence. The extent of the mechanical damage could have established the seriousness of the assault. A third patient had assaulted some ninety Asians and had eventually killed one. It was a type of race war and had been explained as colour prejudice. He confided in me that a friend had been charged as his accomplice and was doing life in prison though he was in no way guilty. A fourth patient stabbed a woman in a toilet and had been interviewed under suspicion of being the Yorkshire Ripper. The Yorkshire Ripper was himself sent to Broadmoor. This patient was very pleasant to talk to and would sit in the dining room playing chess with a computer. He came across as very stable, normal and agreeable and his offence was out of character. There were two or three others who had done very little and one had already been told his transfer to an outside hospital was being arranged. He had just forged a cheque. It was that type of patient I concluded who brought down the average stay of patients in Broadmoor to a matter of years rather than decades. One patient who had killed his mother and two little cousins had also been told he would be discharged in a short time. He didn't believe what he had been told and likewise I seriously started to doubt the little that had been hinted about a quick discharge for me. Only the petty offenders acted as if they would not be doing a long time.

It was about this time that I myself had my first taste of violence in Broadmoor. It was during a meal time and I was occupying a table with two other patients near the service hatch. I started to talk about Evelyn Waugh's autobiography, A Little Learning and of a schoolmaster friend at an awful prep school where he taught for a year. After an outing with the boys to the slopes of Snowden the junior masters were bemoaning the miseries of the day when Waugh's schoolmaster friend confessed to having enjoyed himself very much indeed. When asked what he could possibly have found to enjoy he replied:

"Knox minor. I felt the games a little boisterous so I took Knox minor away behind some rocks. I removed his boot and stocking, opened my trousers, put his dear little foot there and experienced the most satisfying emission."

It as at this point that one of my table companions leapt out of his chair closing his hands round my throat. Although he was not small it was no problem prising his hands apart and releasing myself. But the interesting thing about the whole affair was not that he had attacked me, I myself did not take the matter too seriously, but the reaction of the staff. They made out I had provoked the patient and made me move to another table. I gathered that the patient had been homosexually raped as a child, had developed a hatred of homosexuals and gone out and stabbed one to death. The other chap at the table was the one who had been homosexually raped and held at chisel point in the hospital and he wasn't bothered. Had the roles been reversed I would have been put in seclusion or sent to Norfolk house.

At this point the patient whom I had met on my first full day reached the end of his tether and he contemplated a means of suicide. He had a friend who was good at electronics to advise him and wired himself up to an alarm clock with a timing device designed to go off at the hour and minute of his choice, switch on a current and pump the requisite number of volts through him. He plugged himself into the mains and attempted to go to sleep. Unfortunately he just woke up with a nasty shock.

A patient who strung himself up by the belt of his trousers in the bathroom was successful in his suicide attempt but despite all I battled onto the summer without trying to get over the wall or hang myself and to try and find an escape or oblivion that way. Now that it was summer there was cricket down at the field on Wednesday and Saturday afternoons and evenings. There was also tennis and bowls though I usually just lay on the grass and sunbathed when I went down to the games field. The bright weather that had replaced the terrible grey of winter, did serve to lift my spirits a little. Though there were no film shows during the summer months unlike the winter months, I did now have the opportunity to go to the airing court at Lancaster house. Walking through Lancaster house I commented on the thick studded doors as we passed along the ground floor corridor:

"Why should the doors be so thick?"

"This is a mental hospital" replied the nurse.

The strength needed to break down a door of that thickness would have been an effort for Sampson. There was a hint of the dark ages where inmates were treated like this I felt.

The mere presence of females sitting on a bench in quiet contemplation or hobnobbing in a corner or the nurses with their blue dresses whirling round their legs provided a welcome change from the company of men. But nothing could truly make an indefinite fate in Broadmoor bearable.

Yet there were still my parents who remained a lifeline to me and unable to face seeing me so cowed and miserable they took the opportunity to see Dr. U. They had seen him the previous winter but were still anxious for some reassurance particularly about how long I would do. Dr. U. hinted that I wouldn't be "old and grey" when I was discharged but neither did he leave them with any major hopes about my future prospects.

The one good thing was that I was no longer on drugs. I had repeatedly asked to be taken off them because living with the side effects had been rather unpleasant and as the drugs had no beneficial effects on my mental state, being on them was an unjustifiable intervention. But if being taken off them had in one way been a positive step there was nothing now except my unread summary (though I had still been too close to events to see truly how wronged I had been) that might provide a doctor with a guarantee I'd be safe if freed. Despite my continuous ruminating about getting out and the miseries of Broadmoor I was no nearer the gate than when I had arrived.

At this time our group had sex education and this was to be the start of my treatment from my point of view. Sex education consisted of a series of three films, the first two on contraception and marriage. The third was more interesting and was held in the dayroom where all the patients in my group had gathered sitting in armchairs facing a screen. A nurse operated the projector and the film opened with a sequence about lesbians. Two women returned home from the park and proceeded to make love. There was an emphasis on cleanliness and grooming. The second sequence was of a homosexual couple. One of the partners was doing the ironing which he abandoned when he and his companion decided to make love. This restricted itself to fellatio. The patient who had been homosexually raped as a child tensed up in his chair and bellowed: "I'm not going to watch that." The sequence was entirely innocuous. The third sequence showed a man and a woman on a patch of grass

186

adjacent to a wood, a motorbike propped up nearby. The man was rubbing her breasts up and down with the palm of his hand. They rose, climbed on the bike and zoomed off. They were seen again next to a swimming pool. The man was lying on top of the woman, his arms outstretched, his whole body weight bearing down on her as if driving her into the ground in an act of male domination. To me it clearly symbolised the master slave relationship.

After the film we were all asked how we enjoyed each of the sequences .I felt more fear than pleasure over the heterosexual sequence. The lovemaking had been more like an act of barbarism than a expression of caring. It left me feeling very inadequate and depressed.

Only one patient owned up to liking the sequence on the homosexual couple but the sex education programme did leave me with food for thought.

A male nurse came up to me a little later in the corridor and said: "Have you considered you might be homosexual?" He added that my picking up a gun was a sign of psychological emasculation and that the gun was simply an "extension of the penis." I had felt emasculated but more than that I had felt disfigured. But I knew that if I was prepared to look low enough there would still be someone for me though to find that someone in Broadmoor would be hard. But accepting those who would accept me would be a problem. The female patients in Broadmoor were on average a lot less pretty than the girls I had been out with outside and I explained to the nurse that in the past I had tended to fall for those who were exceptionally good-looking.

I later went to speak to another nurse about my doubts. The nurse was one of the friendliest and kindest on the ward and also knew something about life. He replied:

"Of course you will be able to fall in love. It does not matter what the woman looks like. She need only have one leg. One day you will meet someone who you will be able to love and who will love you."

They were simple words, but the nurse, by being careful not to pervert my words, had not only come up with the right answer, the answer I had had an inkling of in "Carmarthen General Hospital" when I met Barbara, but had given me the vital reassurance I was after. It was really just a question of direction though at that moment it appeared that though I liked all women, a strong self-sufficient woman might not only give me relief from loneliness but hope of love. What worries I had on that score straightaway left me. I was a changed person. But authority remained a threat. It stood over me with the aspect of a giant ready to stamp on me at a whim. Though the poison of Enid's words might have left my system I still felt that I had authority to contend with.

As Broadmoor was referred to as a hospital I decided to see if having effected a recovery I had earned my discharge. I attempted to explain my recovery to the nursing staff hoping they would in turn get the message through to the doctors. However I found few nurses prepared to listen and even fewer to take my words seriously. In the end I was tragically just accused of rationalization.

Meanwhile the doctors continued with their own programme of therapy for me and much later during my time in Broadmoor I was taken off the group I was on and put on a mixed therapy group where I again attempted to explain my recovery.

This group was again held in the dayroom and four or five carefully selected females were brought over from the female wing. They were chosen from amongst the more desirable females in Broadmoor and the males on the group included the triple killer and one of the psychopaths who I had seen with a pretty female patient at the first Christmas party. The male patient was to form a romantic liaison with a girl on the group who once thought she was Joan of Arc leading her to set alight to herself. She was one of the prettiest of the female patients.

As well as talking about my recovery on the group I attempted to talk about such things as man in relation to God and man in relation to the lower animals. I said that God seemed to have nothing to offer but when observing the animals I had come up with a few answers. I added that man was simply a highly evolved type of ape and human nature was akin to that of many lower animals. I tried to move onto a discussion about homosexuality and lesbianism. I was not worried on that score; I just wanted a few guidelines on how I should conduct myself sexually should I be discharged. The male psychopaths on the group, who were completely at sea when I spoke, kept on interrupting. And though the female therapist on the group was in accord when I said couples should complement each other, the doctor did not give me any sign of encouragement. I was to realise that as good, the suppressive personalities that made up much of authority, did not like me.

After a session I did receive a letter from a girl on the group. She said that she was very impressed by what I had to say and went as far as to invite me to a dance organised on behalf of the choral group of which she was a member. I was pleased that at least she understood and I suspected that she had been through the same spiritual struggle as me. She was reasonably good looking with auburn hair and a well-covered body that at least pleased me. But I thought it might be inadvisable after what I had seen in the film shows to be seen with a woman who was not both fragile and weak physically. I also did not want to open myself up to the possibility of rejection.

Shortly after this I was taken off the group "for a rest". It was becoming clear to me that whenever I did begin to broach the real issues of my case there would always be an attempt to confuse the issue or muzzle me. Though there were patients who said it was only after a fair amount of time that they came to realise Broadmoor was a hospital rather than a prison, the end result of this approach towards me was that during the entire time of my involvement with the psychiatric profession, I never did receive any acknowledged treatment for anything I might have complained of.

Soon I began to feel I was not going to be discharged despite my recovery. I had been in Broadmoor well over eighteen months and it took a year usually to wade through the red tape to effect a discharge making a total of well over two years. The hints that I would do a short time were wildly optimistic or misguided as far as I could see. Not only had I found myself but I had tried to fit in with the doctors rather farfetched ideas about me and so keep everyone happy. Beyond that I was not sure what I could do in the way of persuading the doctors that whatever way you looked at it I was ready for discharge. In myself I was not happy about being confined under section 65 and there remained this deep pit of despair whatever the mask I might have worn. And all too often I had this vision of Dr. U., who was already grey and wizened, throwing in his gown and retiring, leaving me stranded in Broadmoor. So I hatched a plan of escape.

CHAPTER 13
A BID FOR FREEDOM.

My plan of escape was far from conventional. I was not going to try and get over the wall which in the end would just have given the police an excuse to slap further charges on me. As soon as I picked up the shotgun I had in effect given the police and everyone else an excuse to get me charged with four major offenses and to break the law in trying a conventional escape would just serve to provoke the wrath of the higher powers. I also knew that writing to MP's, MIND or other bodies would, as said only irritate the higher powers, and I was frightened of the risk of doing longer by getting individuals and organisations from the outside to bring pressure to bear. But as it seemed that I had only started my punishment I still had this feeling that I had nothing to lose. I believed that if I could somehow set the cleverer nurses alight with fiery indignation over the injustices I had suffered I could start a conflagration that would consume the whole hospital, a conflagration that would do damage to the credibility of those with the power to release me unless they acted promptly and did just that. The way to do this seemed to be to get my point across to the nurses in a fashion that could not fail to make them take note. As all letters were so carefully vetted by the censor, himself a nurse, and as important mail was photocopied and often passed to the ward nurses or the doctors, I thought that by sending important information through the censor, I could get my point across. I decided to state my case in a letter to my solicitor (I now had a new solicitor who was significantly a writer and with whom I had not communicated directly before). I had found out that you were allowed to write to the Queen, the Archbishop of Canterbury or your solicitor without having your letter censored if you simply stated on the envelope that you were doing so. I deliberately planned to make no mention of exactly whom I was writing to so that the contents of the letter would be noted and fed back to the doctors and nurses. I planned to word the letter very politely and to make it appear that the revelation of my frame-up was a pure accident. The letter went as follows.

"Dear Mr Grant,

I am now taking the opportunity to introduce myself.

I have improved considerably since my arrival in Broadmoor due to my improved conditions, to a small amount of constructive counselling which has improved my outlook immeasurably, and to the fact that the unpleasant events on my unsettled condition leading to my "offence" and those finally leading to my being sent to Broadmoor are now somewhat distant. However I am still suffering from certain of the consequences of all that has happened one being that it is proving very difficult to present a clear picture of myself. The police statements on the whole painted a rather exaggerated and farfetched picture of everything, even if they succeeded in their aim of presenting a picture of an extreme psychotic breakdown, be the picture false. And it is futile to even try and disagree with what has been alleged. Being in Broadmoor where I am so exposed and vulnerable makes disagreeing even more difficult. Occasionally I have agreed with people purely to avoid further confrontation. But now, when it comes to trying to help myself which can only be done effectively by engaging the assistance of those trained to help, it becomes rather pointless when the latter are working from the wrong premises or in instances from wrong interpretations of events. It is easy just to let the situation continue and blame everything true and false on an illness. But to be run down consistently about my ability to form relationships is achieving nothing. And as I recover from the deep depression that has dogged me on and off for many months, I am beginning to see the situation even more clearly and I wish in a small way stop any further harmful effects of it. I must now refer again to the mode in which the police statements were made...I was to conclude from my first reading of them that it had been effectively decided that to avoid injury to other peoples' reputations and for other minor personal reasons I should be made to appear completely out of control of my thoughts, emotions and actions. I was to be deprived of my rights and credibility. It was now that the word paranoid was introduced, something I had tried to guard against particularly as regards my nose. Only the unfortunate, unplanned and incriminating turn of events when Enid rushed out at me when I went up to the landing outside her room with the gun, worried me...I had been prepared to do a justified spell in prison on the basis of the truth. But in my now unenviable predicament I do not like being attacked everytime I accuse someone of misconduct and I do not like the suggestion that I am a liar when the true liars escape Scot free... Though Broadmoor is not too bad in many ways I don't know that I would not now prefer the outside. Could you please forward Julie's letter to Mr Griffiths,

> Yours faithfully,
> Andrew Robinson.

Before I sent the letter I left it on the chest of drawers in my room for any observant nurse to read. No doubt a nurse did read it for a little later I was asked to see Dr. U. in the charge nurse's office where both the charge nurse and Dr. U. tried to make out in veiled terms that I would not be locked up for too much longer. Obviously the letter might have been embarrassing for a few people. But I didn't have complete faith in anyone anymore.I had heard of patients who had been told years previously that they would be getting out soon and nothing had happened. Dr. U. was reasonably reliable in comparison with many doctors but I had personally only known one patient from the ward to be discharged and I knew that if certain documents of questionable veritude were allowed to remain unquestioned I would be written down as a monster for all time. Anyway I could not tell anymore whether people were just "jollying" me along or whether they were being genuinely honest. I resolved to send the letter.

After I had sent it I spoke to a very pleasant nurse, a Times crossword wizard, in the airing court during exercise. I told him that before going up to Enid's room with the gun I stuffed my pockets full of cartridges with the intention, not of hurting anyone, but of drawing as much attention to myself as possible. "You certainly did that" he replied and he seemed to comprehend exactly what I was trying to say. I now had a worthwhile ally in the nurse; even so I did begin to regret having sent the letter for I feared that the reaction that might ensue could be dangerous for me.

A little after I had posted the letter I received a couple of admiring glances from nurses in the ward. The nurse whom I had spoken to on the airing court even said in the charge nurse's office one day that the letter was "a brilliant idea". After that other nurses, some whom I hardly knew, said "Hello Andrew" and smiled in a way that they had never done before. I attributed the whole new attitude to my letter and I was pleased that people at last seemed to be taking notice of my plight, even though I was nervous of too wide-spread a reaction.

I decided to try and back up my assertions by doing the work that previous solicitors had failed to do and I wrote off to two people at St.David's University College who did witness my actions through my year at Lampeter and whom I thought could give a more accurate and reliable account of me. One was Steve, the other David. My letter to Steve was a straightforward request for information of a general nature. My letter to David angled at getting more specific information about events. Unfortunately the letter was not direct enough and pandered too much to the Broadmoor set-up. I also called Lorna poisonous because of her prank, masterminded by Enid, to ruin my reputation during my first term at Lampeter and though I was actually very fond of Lorna and thought highly of her, the words were bound to lead some nurses to think.

Despite a delay in receiving replies to my letters and despite the absence of any word about a discharge I kept my head.

Then a letter did arrive from David asking if he should go ahead and send the information at his disposal. He had little conception of the reality of my situation and wrongly assumed that I was allowed home at weekends. In normal circumstance I would have replied to David's letter but nurses on the ward had started in many subtle ways to apply pressure on me and it was also suggested

192

that I had gone far enough and that to go any further would be to overstate my case. Tragically I did not reply to David's offer of information and consequently it never came.

Four weeks after I had sent the letter to Steve, his reply arrived on the ward. It was evening when I received it. What happened was that a nurse called me into the charge nurse's office and with his face beaming brightly presented me with the letter. It had a Lampeter postmark on it and the censor had pencilled on the envelope the letters R.M.O. (responsible medical officer).The letter had been sent by the censor directly to Dr. U. and I could tell from the date on the postmark that he had retained it for three weeks. When I took the letter out of the envelope I found it said in part what I wanted to hear, that the incident with the shotgun outside Enid's room had to be seen in the light of a suicide attempt and that as with my other suicide attempts I had been talking happily to people beforehand suggesting that in all three instances I was not out of control and that I had really been attention seeking. He had said enough and I viewed the letter as a victory for justice.

Then at some point round now the copy of Julie's letter to Mr Griffiths arrived from my new solicitors. Only now did I discover that she had simply described the fantasies of the prosecution witnesses. When in desperation I had picked up the shotgun in Tony's room a month into the summer term at Lampeter it had been exaggerated to mean I had threatened to kill Enid. Julie gave as justification the ragging over my nose in public but in fact I had not wanted to hurt Enid, only get my point across and there had been no ragging up to that point. When I showed it to a nurse in the charge nurse's office he did point out that the accusations were made up. He put it in my file--ideally I would have liked it burned.

But now the pressure really started. The first instance of this was when a nurse walked into the dayroom and said to me: "You'll do thirty years." I assumed that because I did not have the information at David's disposal my words had as usual, been distorted, exaggerated and taken out of context and that a body of the nurses or even the doctors had believed the plausible liars who had only been out for misguided vengeance and poured scorn on the truth. I didn't ignore the possibility that the threat might also have just been a joke at my expense, a sick joke like telling someone their children had been killed in a car crash, and after a natural display of annoyance, I had not yet been struck down by fear, I went and asked another nurse how long I would do. "A few more weeks" he replied.

A nurse came into the dayroom and said to me: "You'll never get out. "I suddenly felt frightened. I knew the terrible danger of being misrepresented and guessed I might have been depicted in a bad light. I went to see a kindly charge nurse and asked him if

193

anything was happening about me."We can let you out" he replied. "But if you reoffend you will do much longer." The charge nurse cited the case of another patient who had run a sword through someone and who had been discharged because he had made out he was normal, but had allegedly reoffended. I hadn't been trying to say I had been totally unaffected by the things that had happened to me; I was just objecting to gross injustice and gross misrepresentation.

The bad attitude of nurses continued and in reacting to it I was considered "high". Soon I began to regret the letter to my new solicitor and after a few weeks, having heard nothing more about a discharge, I wished I had just carried on the farce. Indeed my increasing fear over the situation soon made me very depressed. What I did not consider at the time was that I was being tested. When authority tested someone it tried to induce a nervous breakdown and one of my friends on the ward who had seen this happen before said that he had no genuine liking for the doctors responsible. Tony had himself been warned by a doctor to be careful unless he wanted him to walk all over him with his "big hobnail boots". But I couldn't think what authority would or could achieve by hurting me in my most vulnerable area other than to get me to say what it wanted to hear.

After some weeks of unremitting anguish a nurse again tried to suggest to me that I was homosexual. I had had much varying advice from different quarters and this nurse was I'm sure just tying to help. But whatever you had or had not done, the doctors could for genuine or non-genuine motives,justify your detention in Broadmoor if they could pin a label on you. The label might refer to a psychiatric illness or to a personality disorder. To be in hospital and to escape being labelled as normal people who had engineered their admission into a hospital for research reasons had found, was impossible, and homosexuality was a recognised personality disorder in the eyes of some. The advice led my thoughts astray and did nothing to help my case.

The attitude of some nurses was soon such that my depression became dire. Only in Cardiff Jail had I felt as bad. I was truly being torn on the mental rack. Then I received another letter from my middle-aged English master. As we had developed a mutual respect I valued him as a correspondent particularly in my present unhappy circumstances. But in my reply I feared that I had made my misery and desperation apparent. I had felt that in betraying my emotions, I had destroyed his remaining faith in me. Because of my dire misery I did not have the grasp on life to even compose a decent letter. The institution and its operators had completely got to me. That was my last letter to him.

One night at "banging up" time the night nurses just ignored me as my side-room was locked. Normally they made some sort of acknowledgement. I had reached the bottom of my fortunes. I was dirt. Suddenly I felt all the anxiety, emotion and fight drain out of me. That night I almost resigned myself to never getting out.

However the next day the fight started again. What was still the matter? Why did people react to me the way they did? Why in my hour of need had they turned round and gone out to destroy me instead of rallying to my support? Why were they always so eager to condemn? The accusation of paranoia nonsense. The persecution was real. After all I had been placed in Broadmoor without limit of time on the basis of an excuse and John had specifically stated he hoped to see me locked in four thick walls for the rest of my days.

I thought about other acts of persecution in my life, being teased and also bullied on that one occasion at senior school. I had not looked upon this as persecution at the time but such treatment was designed to make life miserable. But it was being framed and sent to Broadmoor as a paranoid that got to me.

I considered that deep down in my personality structure there might still be something wrong. Monkeys always turned on the weak or defenceless members of the troop. Was I considered a burden or a liability? If I could fathom out what was wrong I could put it right. Even persuade the staff to recommend my discharge.

I concluded that though I had had a couple of perhaps angry moments I was just too moral. I thought that a strong aggressive woman might complement me though I was in fact attracted to all types of women, even weak ones, and no doubt lay somewhere in between the two poles of violent and non violent.

I began to reflect on the violent aspect of sex. What was the connection if any? Some of the male patients were sexually excited by violence. So were many in society outside. There were women who liked to be hit around by their husbands. There were men who liked to be whipped and stamped on by women in uniform. Was that perversion or just an extension of the domination submission principle outlined in sex therapy. At any event the trend of thinking in the hospital was that violence was a component of sex and a film shown in the Central Hall called The Corpse Wore Satin starring Marlon Brando backed this assertion. It specifically said that men were evil and sadistic and women good and masochistic. This was demonstrated in a bondage scene in the film where the heroine was tied to a bedpost. Was I, a largely non violent individual, to reverse these two roles?

Through masturbation I set about finding out where I stood sexually. Was I predominantly male or female in outlook? I was entering a period of deep spiritual darkness. For the first time I questioned seriously the moral basis of my thinking. I was groping around for meaning and the answers. I assumed that in the normal pattern of thinking, women, who were usually physically and

195

mentally weaker than men, were only happy when submitting, being abased like a slave, while the male, the hunter and protector, was happier dominating. Opposite attract. Love would only follow once harmony had been achieved. But I was aware even now of pressures being placed upon me and my comments and observations being dismissed by the staff. I believed I was on the right track but my endless searchings for the truth were just dismissed as lunatic manifestations. In fact I was to see that I was good and strong and that you could be bad and weak and I needed a strong good woman.

Meanwhile I went off at a tangent. If they were going to reduce me I would not resist but abase myself instead. I was not the only one to descend into the abyss. There was a patient who imagined himself as a monk licking the dirt off floors or of being the victim of a gang rape. He fashioned realistic and accurately shaped dildoes in the carpentry shop smuggling them up to the ward, a larger one each week. These he would insert up his rectum. To a limited extent I copied him. I even sustained marginal anal damage. It took five years to be turned into a homosexual and many had experimented with it. One patient spoke of his experience of pederasty with excrement splashing all over the toilet floor. I tried to think like a homosexual and later even experimented very briefly with Tony, but in the process I got very tensed up physically. I knew I was not in any way abnormal in my leanings but the medical authorities seized their chance and I was informed that though I had been off drugs for six months, I was being put back on them, the usual way you were told you were mad or stepping out of line. The largactil only succeeded in killing off the remainder of my dwindling store of aggression. I had been chemically tamed and it was as if the last nail had been hammered into my coffin.

I decided to speak about my predicament to a patient on the ward who was doing a degree with the Open University.

"It does not matter what I say or do I am always in the wrong" I said.

"You're not in Broadmoor because you're mad" he replied. "You're mad because you're in Broadmoor."

"So what do I do about it?"

"Love big brother. Love big brother and he will love you."

What I had most feared deep down had been succinctly put. A consultant psychiatrist was like a god in a very real sense. For many patients their only hope lay in remembering this fact and then fitting in with their doctor, god, the supreme being, Big Brother. He said who and what you were. It was even his prerogative to rewrite your past. And as for truth and justice; well such things were just the product of the moral imagination. Doctors dealt with humanity in its raw primitive state. I might have thought of myself as the true victim and Enid simply as the alleged victim. But the fact that Enid had the brute strength of the law on her side and now that brute strength had had its way everything else was irrelevant. I had been mistaken to place so much emphasis on truth and justice. Such things were not often part of the real world. But what was real was that Broadmoor was the "lavatory of society" and that I was now a lump of shit. It would be unsavoury for any doctor to come and fish me out from amongst the other turds.

My only hope of escape was to play ball with the system. No, more than that, sell my soul. To escape the ingeniously woven web that ensnared me I would have to say, think and do exactly what the system wanted. I determined that I would cooperate as much as was sensible and instead of protesting when I was put back on drugs, the side effects of which were colossal, I said that I felt much better on them and I did not mention getting out again. I made it seem that I agreed with everything that had been alleged about me in Broadmoor and after a discussion with a nurse, asked if I could join the part one City and Guilds Electronics class to suggest I was at least stable enough to study. I then sat down to wait for my discharge and though I hoped I would not have to wait more than five years I did not dismiss the thought that I might have to wait twenty five. I knew that I now simply had to leave my future in the hands of the doctors.

At around this time I spoke to a fellow bookbinder who had been an ambulance driver before his arrest, about possible methods of suicide. Although my depression in Broadmoor was three or four times more intense than it had been outside, the result of seeing my future eclipsed, I could be perfectly controlled and having argued away the logicality of attempting suicide in a place like Broadmoor, had withstood the extremes of mental pain. Now I was looking out for effective ways of committing suicide because I knew that I could not continue to live with the terrible uncertainty of my situation and had at least to contemplate all possible ways out of it. I considered stabbing myself in the neck with one of the knives resting in the tray on the bench and asked the patient to point out the main arteries. He indicated where the carotid artery was and I could feel it throbbing with my finger. I considered that by ridding myself of the uncertainty I could come to an acceptance of my situation. But acceptance was difficult to achieve and meanwhile I just held on. The only other suicidal idea I had was to throw a television that was connected to the mains into a bath full of water and electrocute myself.

But two or three nurses speaking to me on the subject of my mental health did give me much encouragement expressing the view that I was getting on well on drugs and though that wasn't true I began to feel more secure. And at least it was better to be withdrawn than aggressive for an aggressive attitude was always considered the worst thing in Broadmoor even if it was the result of wrongful imprisonment.

The next summer my parents arranged to see Dr. U. during a visit to me. I sat in the visiting hall glancing up at the clock on the wall watching the minutes go by as I eagerly awaited their return. Did they have any good news to report? At last the figures of my mother and father appeared in the doorway of the visiting hall. They sat down. I asked my father how the interview went. He was beaming brightly. He said that he had as usual asked when I would be let out. "Well, he won't be old and grey" Dr. U. had replied as always. "What if we go back to South Africa?" "If you go back to South Africa I could arrange for a conditional discharge for Andrew to South Africa" were Dr. U.'s words.

My dream had come true. Everything I had worked for had finally born fruit. However I was to assume when I heard the news that in order to effect a patient's discharge in Britain, not only the doctor's recommendation was needed but a consensus amongst the medical staff. As someone with a vicarage ideology was not liked by certain people in authority and I had thus been written off, consensus was difficult. But I could go abroad provided Dr. U gave his backing and the Home Secretary consented. And if in the end Dr. U. had based a few of his opinions of me on what people ill-disposed to me had said, he had at least come round to the view that I was not dangerous and now at least recognised my ability to survive, which reflected an honest mind on his part.

When I was informed by my parents of what Dr. U. had said I agreed with them that the wisest thing at this juncture would be to return to South Africa and my father decided to give three months notice to his bishop.

News soon spread that I was going back to South Africa. It was always an occasion of excitement when a patient was told that he would be discharged or transferred to an outside hospital and I felt excited as well. Though the enormous pressure had suddenly been taken off me, I remained careful, for just a little while before, Tony, who had been informed he was to be transferred to an outside hospital, went and hit a patient over the head with a snooker cue and had been transferred to the refractory block instead.

My parents and sister soon set about trying to establish themselves in South Africa while I continued to try and make the most of Broadmoor. By some luck I had passed part one City and Guilds Electronics and I did not feel deserted by my parents for my father had promised that he would come back to England if I had not been discharged within the time stated by Dr. U..

It was March 1981. I had been told I would be in South Africa by then. March was the date my father had promised to come back should my discharge be blocked or delayed. I told a nurse of

198

the situation and he mentioned my discharge to Dr. U. who said he would write off a letter straightaway. I had been afraid that nothing would happen, that Dr. U. would retire and that I would be left stranded in Broadmoor. But my father did return to England. I was waiting on the staircase for a visit to see him with Tony when Tony suddenly made a grab for my testicles. The most embarrassing part was that a nurse was viewing the proceedings through the glass peephole in the main door to Somerset one and the incident was very hard to explain away. My father took the opportunity to see Dr. U. who just reassured him and advised him to return to South Africa. It emerged that there had been problems and that I could not be admitted into South Africa straight from a special hospital. I was told I would have to spend three months in an open hospital first. It was part of a long stalling procedure on the part of the South African authorities who were determined not to allow ex-mental patients into South Africa but would neither say "yay" or "nay" to my entry. My father returned to South Africa.

I had to see a young female psychologist about my discharge. We sat down together in the interview room along with a trainee psychologist. I presented her with some photographs of myself before and after as I wanted it established that I had at no time been deluded and that I was not as good-looking now. I spoke of people being graded by their looks but that by lowering my standards I could fit. She hadn't the intelligence to understand and maliciously concluded that because I had shown her photographs of myself I must still be worried about my appearance. And though she seemed very pleasant I later discovered she had written a dreadful, dishonest report calculated to keep me in Broadmoor. Time and time again people with influence would only look at the bad things, most of which were their imaginings, and though Dr. U. was pressing for my discharge in this country she was responsible for my parents having to remain in South Africa. She got on better with the more aggressive types like the homosexual killer whom she was very fond of because he had killed.

I was told I was to be seen by a Dr. Pears from Exeter about my transfer. My heart leapt. She I hoped might have a better understanding of my case because of what my father had told her three years previously. She came up to Broadmoor with a female social worker, a male charge nurse and a female registrar. Their attitude at the start clearly indicated how influenced they had been by the lies in the police statements and by the farfetched psychiatric reports, but I nevertheless tried to make my point as cogently as I could and Dr. Pears did agree to have me as a patient for a period of three months. Freedom was now a real possibility.

At approximately this time I was put on depot injections or depixol and taken off oral medication. Though I hated injections they were a good sign for they meant I was being prepared for transfer. I still regarded drugs as a form of poisoning but if by taking them the doctors were kept happy, that was the main thing. Had I been able to adjust the medication myself it might have helped. But whatever the dosage of largactil it was too much, in effect suppressing all aggression in an already under-aggressive person. The end result was a zombie.

Before I left a television station decided to do a short series on Broadmoor as part of an evening programme and a reporter and television team went through the hospital interviewing patients and staff, filming the various aspects of hospital life. The case of Gary Jackson was cited. He had bought a spade. Dr. Tidmarsh explained on the television that his confinement on those grounds would not make sense unless you understood it was to "do in" his father and mother. As it was he didn't harm any one and he explained to me that he had been pushed down the stairs and every bone in his body had been broken by his father. I was captured on a few seconds of footage striding along the terrace with the rest of the group from the shops in a lumberjacket.

Shortly before I left an adolescent patient came up to me in the dining room and said that he had had an affair with another patient whom he had met in the shops and that he had given the patient a gold ring. The recipient of the ring had then terminated the relationship and the adolescent patient was very confused and upset. I told him not to worry adding that the ring could be recovered. The adolescent patient's hero was Frank Mitchell, the mad axeman, and he had come to believe that the answer to everything was violence. The following day he attacked a patient in the tailors stabbing him repeatedly in the neck and shoulders. His victim was a very meek and unassuming individual. I was told that the adolescent patient had been talking of killing me. I said nothing. Though people had told the worst lies to get me natural life I did not react the same way and did not think of going out of my way to get the adolescent patient condemned even if he would have to face the full processes of the law.

The day of my transferral came. It was mid 1981. The previous night I had packed all my books and belongings and the following morning David helped me carry my bags to the waiting taxi which would take me to Exe Vale Hospital in Exeter. I was accompanied by two nurses in plain clothes, one in front and one in the back. This time there were no handcuffs. As I passed through the gates of the hospital I breathed a sigh of relief. It was the first time I had been outside those gates for two years and ten months. I had escaped the nightmare. But to escape had involved many compromises. It had involved the total sacrifice of my dignity. It had involved denying the truth in my favour and it seemed that only by a fluke had I escaped. It had been a question of knowing which "horse" to back and to know what he wanted. Of course there had been the sacrifice made by my parents, their cost and sacrifice in terms of money, pain, effort and persistence. But I was now out of it. Of course I was still in the power of the Home Office in the same way that a prisoner who has served his period of a life sentence in prison. I was not entirely my own master. I had to go and stay wherever the Home Office said and I could be hauled back within those grim walls at any time. Unless I could legally escape the shores of England which was still my ultimate ambition.

CHAPTER 14
A PALE DAWN.

I was at last free but I felt freed not so much from my physical chains as from the recurrent mental anguish that prison and Broadmoor had induced. Freedom did not come to me as a great jolt. There is often talk about rehabilitation and to a limited extent that might be sensible for someone who has been locked away for very many years but I had been inside for a comparatively short while and the world I was coming out to had changed little from when I had last seen it.

On the journey to Exe Vale the taxi stopped at a motorway service station cafe. We all went inside to buy a cup of coffee and this involved handling money which I hadn't done for years for in prison and Broadmoor everything had been done on paper and though I enjoyed handling money I don't wish to overstate it. It was however both strange and wonderful to be amongst ordinary people again and to feel a part of their world, the world I had been drawn away from with so much anguish and reluctance. Total freedom would not have been to great a step for me though that is not to say I minded the presence of the nurses at the motorway cafe or that I thought of them as infringing on my freedom.

But for one more stop the rest of the journey to Exe Vale was swift and uneventful. The hospital at Wonford, one of three belonging to the Exe Vale trio, was an imposing building of grey stone set in extensive grounds and looked more like a country house than a hospital. I later caught some Americans photographing it as if it was a National Trust property to show their friends back home. The car was directed to a side entrance and I was admitted to a newly decorated ward with comfortably furnished rooms called the Bucknill centre. The Broadmoor nurses left and I was consigned to the care of something approaching ordinary nurses, both male and female.

"Christ, I thought I would be on a locked ward" I said.

"This is a locked ward" replied a female nurse.

It might have been a locked ward but there were no bars on the windows, there was no suggestion of security except for the locked door and I did not feel at all trapped or closed in. There were also female patients on the ward which was a relief as I assumed I had been put away to deliberately remove me from the company of women.

A female nurse made an inventory of all my belongings. She was young and pretty. I no doubt found her prettier than I would otherwise have done having been deprived of female company for so long. I was touched by her gentle manner and femininity which struck me as how nurses should be and ran in contrast to the gruffness I had encountered in Broadmoor from many of the nurses.

After the inventory had been made the nurse showed me to my room. It was in every sense a bedroom as opposed to a cell and the bed had been beautifully made with fresh clean sheets, thick blankets and a coverlet. There was a dressing table, an armchair, a bedside table and beside light. In my room I placed my bags.

"Are the doors locked at night?" I asked.

"No, of course not" replied the nurse in a surprised voice.

A little later the nurse left and I settled into my bedroom for a good rest. This I was allowed to do. The combination of nerves and my new surroundings had tired me.

Lunch came. It took place in a dining room in the open section of the ward. The quality of food was a great improvement on Broadmoor but I was unable to eat. I was able to drink though and what I had to drink was something I had never been offered in Broadmoor, orange juice.

That afternoon I saw a Dr. Hudson. I found that for the first time in over three years I was under no pressure and I was able to speak freely to a doctor. Dr. Hudson, who it appeared had no notes on me, took it all very informally perched on the edge of a desk in the interview room. I spoke to him of certain of my problems and obsessions and how they had fitted in with my ideas about life. I explained how my outlook had changed and how I had changed. Afterwards he said to a nurse he would send me back to South Africa now if he had his way.

That night was one of sublime peace. It was incredible to me that there were real women sleeping and dreaming one or two doors away from me. Or that if I wanted to urinate I didn't have to resort to a chamber pot but could just walk out of my door to the toilet at the end of the passage. The previous night I had been a life prisoner in Britain's most notorious mental asylum. Now I was a trusted individual again.

Over the next week I was amazed by how friendly everyone continued to be. It was almost as if I was being treated as a human being again. I was called Andrew and the nurses as well as the patients said "please" and "thank you". Civility had been restored. It appeared that on the surface at least I was respected again and the anxiety as it had manifested itself in Broadmoor along with the fear, had gone. I was still a little tense but it was only due to my new surroundings.

A few days after my arrival I had an interview with Dr. Pears. She asked me if I thought had been ill and I declined to answer. I did not want to be drawn into issues where my ideas and the ideas of previous doctors would be in dispute. Besides I assumed that Dr. Hudson, who was present, had done all the explaining that was necessary. The word ill had so many connotations. For example did she mean emotionally disturbed or psychotic? I did not want my understanding of the word to conflict with that of Dr. Pears. The rest of the interview touched upon how I was reacting to my change of environment. At the end of the interview Dr. Pears said she would see me the following Friday and the Fridays after that when she did her ward round. The doctors I discovered were no longer the elusive, distant, deitific beings that they had been in Broadmoor and the relationship between doctor and patient had been restored to something like sense. How I wondered could it be fruitful when a major component of it was fear as in Broadmoor?

Now that I was installed in Exe Vale I thought I should write to all my acquaintances to inform them of my change of address. I took out a letter writing pad and pen, sat down on the edge of my bed and put pen to paper. One person I wrote to was Mr Griffiths saying that I had just effected an imaginary cure to a ridiculous imaginary illness and quietly got over my problems myself. That I hasten to add was no fault of mine but the contortions I had been made to go through. I put the letters in envelopes, stamped and addressed them, then posted them in the post box in the front entrance. I was glad to have happy news to report and expected the recipients to reply.

Coming out into the outside world I had resolved to put into practice all the ideas I had formed regarding my conduct towards the female sex. Having endured a lot of negative experiences I was subdued and undecided as to whether I was dominant or submissive though I was probably stuck somewhere in the middle. But at least my theories made sense and I kept my eyes glued just in case the right person should appear. One female patient I encountered had brown hair, an average build, very pretty features and was called Charlotte. She seemed locked in a world of her own even though she did show a flicker of interest in two or three of the male patients who passed through the ward. Charlotte had threatened to dent in her father's head with a brick and had been put on a section. Compared with most patients she had spent quite a long time on the ward. She was not aggressive or abusive but restless. The boredom of life on a closed ward seemed to have affected her. But though I sensed her restlessness I did not try and pin her down to a conversation. This sprang primarily from my avowal to have nothing more to do with pretty or beautiful women, at least on a serious level. Enid had demonstrated by her conduct that she had a dominant bias and liked dominant men though having had my features slightly damaged I could never have competed with her.

Even if I avoided pretty women neither did I gravitate towards any available Medusa for I did not feel, despite my letdowns in Broadmoor, that any relationship I had with a woman should be crowned with the principle of ugliness. I no longer recoiled from ugliness but neither did I wholeheartedly embrace it. On the ward there was a fat inquisitive girl with a face resembling a gargoyle who used to sit opposite me in an alcove and just stare at me. I displayed an almost cruel indifference towards her which well illustrated my desire to achieve a happy medium and not to suddenly swing from an extreme of beauty to an extreme of ugliness in whom I looked for as a life partner.

During this period I was not restricted entirely to the Extra Care Unit and oneday the sister, who was a woman of some independence, invited me out to play cricket on the spacious lawn in front of the Bucknill centre. Some stumps had been set up and the patients from the main part of the ward had assembled in a circle to field balls hit by the batsman. Although I was not sports mad now, cricket did offer a distraction.

One morning I was asked to attend the community meeting which was held in the ward's principal lounge. We all sat round the edge on chairs with the overflow of nurses and patients curling up on the floor. We started discussing problems with the ward though personal problems were not aired. These meetings were to become a regular thing getting a bit repetitive with patients sitting round like lumps of clay praying for the end to arrive.

I particularly enjoyed it when a female nurse offered to take me into town. To walk into town, to wander down the High street window shopping and to be able to stroll into the clothes and book shops and browse around with complete freedom was a wonderful experience for someone who had been enclosed in a total institution for three years not once having had the opportunity to step out the main gate.

After two weeks I found I had recovered my appetite and started to settle completely into the new regime. But I remained mildly self-conscious and had not yet met anyone with the qualities I was looking for who had shown any great interest in me. I was essentially engaging in a passive experiment seeing how I fitted and where I stood. I simply surmised that if I was to a certain extent ignored it was because I was not as handsome as I used to be. That is not to say I thought of myself as ugly or that I believed I was incapable of forming close relationships.

Despite my doubts I was let out into the main part of the ward after three weeks as a permanent measure. I was given a new bedroom which I had to share and my integration into the hospital community was completed.

I had expected a handful to reply to my letters. I was being over-optimistic. Only three people still thought enough of me to write back. They were Jerome, my former French mistress (and her husband) and my former Biology master. I received a couple of visits and on one occasion my former French mistress even took me out to see a Shakespearean production at the Northcotte. We were standing near the bar at the interval drinks in hand, with numerous smartly attired people milling about the plush interior, when, above the hubbub, I asked her what she had been told about me, notably what I had done to be sent to Broadmoor, an unfair question, but I was curious to know what rumours had been passed around by people like John who hadn't lived far from West Buckland, my old school. She replied that she had been told I had killed a girl. I was thrown into a mood of despondency. I thought of her as being terribly brave to still want to associate with me when under the assumption I was a murderer. When it came to it I hadn't hurt anyone and I was amazed that people dismissed such slander so easily when it resulted in people being wrongly labelled and sent to Broadmoor or the ruination of a reputation. My former French mistress at least still had memories of me as a success and held me in respect despite the ignominy of my having been sent to Broadmoor and the arbitrary labels that accrue to mental patients. But she was unable to comprehend the sudden collapse of my spirits, she was a little wary of me after that and though on discovering the cause of my upset she attempted to deny her words, the evening was spoilt. Though John, one of my best friends, had turned on me in my hour of need committing perjury to get me life in a secure hospital leading me to still question the concept of friendship, I thought I should hang onto the one or two who were still prepared to put themselves out for me.

At this time a new patient arrived on the ward called Steve. He was twenty eight, tall, slim with black hair, reticent and of middle-class background. He had led a withdrawn life and thought the disc jockey Peter Powell, was in his head. He was to share a room with me and once I had got to know him found him congenial company. At this time I started occupational therapy which I found unsatisfying so used to avoid it and walk round the hospital grounds with Steve instead. On these walks we would discuss all manner of things about the hospital or ourselves and we were seen together so much we became known as the terrible twins.

I also got to know Charlotte better. This was the result of having been thrown together. Early on during my stay a trip to Bristol zoo was organised when matters between Charlotte and myself took a different turn. As we stepped out of the coach she asked me to be her "escort". I did not very well feel I could say "no" to such an offer though I had resolved not to read too much into the invitation. The fact that I was hungry for love and affection did not make me a fool but I did feel valued for once. Charlotte and I broke away from the main party and we started to wander about the zoo on our own. We briefly viewed the animals and reptiles though neither of us dwelt on the cages for long. My thoughts were not on cages or even my own previous captivity but the fact that I felt alive again, even though I knew that Charlotte could be no more than a game to me.

Then in the middle of the zoo we found a bar. I hadn't drunk a drop for four years and suddenly the opportunity had presented itself. Charlotte and I entered the bar. I bought a pint of cider and thirstily gulped at it. Charlotte ordered a pint of Guinness and that too disappeared quickly. She was obviously keen on her drink and if she and I did not share many interests, we did in drink. For me though alcohol was now something I treated as fun rather than as a drug. We both ordered refills and went and sat on chairs in the patio outside. Soon I felt quite tipsy. After we had finished our third pint we each went for refills and then relaxed under an oak tree our pint glasses resting on the grass beside us.

We lay side by side very close to one another. Charlotte started to stare into my eyes and I felt my heart melt. Certainly the poetry of a pretty girl so close was as inspiring as any love sonnet I knew. Our lips were a foot apart. It would have been so easy for me to obey my instincts, reach over and kiss her but I remembered my vow not to have anything more to do with pretty women and I turned my head away.

Later, on our way back to the coach, Charlotte asked me if I would like to share a squat with her. I said nothing. A little further on she stooped to pick up a dog end which she proceeded to light and smoke. She had descended a long way I realised. But because she was pretty she could get away with it. Anyway I had to accept the standards of those who would accept me.

I made a few more friends as the weeks went by. In addition I got in touch with the Whitakers. Mr Whitaker was my father's old church warden at Payhembury and they invited me out for the day, a visit that was to be repeated several times. I also saw the Rev. Whitaker who had been friendly with my father and whose children I vaguely knew. I was invited to the rectory. We went blackberry picking in the green wooded countryside near Tiverton. We followed a brambly path and filled three cartons. But though the rector was very warm and amusing, back at the rectory the children, who were about my age, kept their distance. They no doubt saw me as the product of a mental hospital and probably regarded me as infected.

Back at Exe Vale I had more to do with Charlotte. Boredom more than anything wrought this. One evening she invited me to the Flying Horse, a pub down the road, and I went over to the charge nurse's office and wangled permission from the night nurse to go with her. At the bar she ordered a Guinness and I a cider. We sat down at a table and sipped at our glasses. But though it was said Charlotte and I were having a light-hearted affair we hadn't even kissed. My main doubts about our friendship lay in the fact that she was masochistic like many women. The only way to win her over was to be hard and cruel. For example when I said I hated pregnant women she as all over me. All I meant was that their shape displeased me. Charlotte was pregnant I discovered, though not obviously so. We had a few more pints then returned to the hospital. But even with drink inside me I was quite sane and in control and I was careful not to be disorderly or to get carried away. Charlotte and I were to go drinking on other occasions as well which did make life more entertaining and interesting for both.

About a month later, as we were walking through the grounds of the hospital, Charlotte turned to me and asked if I would like to go to London with her for a weekend. I couldn't have gone because I was bound by my section so she went on her own.

On her return she appeared on the ward and came up to me saying: "I've been a naughty girl." In London she had decided to track down the father of her future child and he had actually returned to Exeter with her. Her words were the only acknowledgement she made of any grand underlying sexual passions. I was a little sad but I did not take the blow too hard. I was now ruled by my own sense and intuition, the only ruler I could trust and I had passed my first test since being free. After that I took up with as girl on the ward called Elizabeth.

A further description of Elizabeth is perhaps now necessary for I calculated she was the sort of girl I could enjoy some success with. I was the first to talk to her. She was standing in the alcove off the corridor when I first went up to her and said: "Smoking is a substitute for sex." She always had a cigarette hanging from her mouth. She was small with wavy light hair and reasonably small features. She was very forward and talkative and the medical staff who had a word to describe every mood or gesture, were tempted to call her "high". To me her liveliness and talkativeness were appealing.

On another occasion she grabbed me by the arm and led me round the hospital grounds. I did not have it in mind to go out with her then though the thought of kissing her did cross my mind. And psychologically she seemed to be just what I needed. She did not intimidate me and brought me out of myself. It didn't appear to matter what I said, she took it all in good heart. She was also the most articulate patient on the ward and I needed someone informed like her.

I rarely mentioned Broadmoor during my time in Exe Vale. Certainly I did not to Elizabeth. But I did to Steve. We were walking round the hospital. Our conversation included Charlotte and Elizabeth. Now I decided to bring up Broadmoor. Steve was slow to grasp what I was saying as there were so many "ifs" and "buts" in my descriptions. It was not surprising he did not understand properly or fully. The doctors hadn't. And anyway, who was he, an example of someone who believed because he was being treated he must be benefitting from it (though he was never to recover) to disagree with the doctors treatment of me? But I was constantly dismayed by his misconceptions about me and some of the false conclusions he was beginning to draw about me. He was apt to assume that I had done something far worse than I had admitted to to have been sent to Broadmoor and brushed aside my protests at such suggestions. My punishment was to have been sent to Broadmoor. From that he concluded wrongly that I must have killed someone. I realised it was dangerous to mention Broadmoor to anyone.

The Bucknill centre was a busy ward and including the E.C.A. had about twenty five patients of whom Steve, Charlotte and Elizabeth, are the only ones I have mentioned. People came in for depression, for delusions, for mania, for hysteria and for alcoholism. The aforementioned three were at least controlled.But as indicated not all were. I was sitting in the dining room eating my lunch. There were several patients scattered round the dining room and relative peace reigned. Then a woman with greying streaks in her hair from the E.C.A. clambered upon a table amongst the plates, tomato and brown sauce bottles and started to wave her hands about like a conductor urging us all to sing. We just carried on ignoring her. We just accepted such outbursts of insanity, which in the Bucknill centre, had exceeded anything I had known in Broadmoor, as normal. The woman was probably more suited to Ash ward, a ward for older female patients and was not the only one to stand out by her behaviour. A male patient who was sorely afflicted by voices once dived head first through a plate glass window.

Another patient was rather a ogre in appearance and used to prowl about the ward in a way that made everyone feel ill at ease. He would come up to me and go on about Christianity as if purity and a belief in God were the two things that would render you acceptable to him. He would lambast anyone whom he assumed was not a Christian and it was not in your interests to deny it as you could then expect him to issue threats that could be worrying. The patient juxtaposed his faith with an evident disturbing brutal streak and admitted to having strangled a few cats.

One day I passed the charge nurse's office when I noticed a woman sitting in a chair inside in a nightdress and dressing gown. She had bruises all over her face where she had been beaten by her husband and was an example of someone who was normal but just a victim of her family. Often patients were just the victims of society or their families and it should have been their persecutors rather than them in hospital.

As it was I got on well with most patients and my progress over the months was noticed by the staff. Slowly my drugs were reduced. When I complained of the side effects they were reduced even more. Eventually my depixol injections were reduced from once a week to once a month. But I also had to take a minimum of oral medication namely orap for so-called schizophrenia and kemadrin for the side effects. The Whitakers from Payhembury noticed that with medication reduced I was much more lively and alert. Before people had assumed that I must be abnormal because they could not see the drugs inside me upsetting my general performance. Now I appeared more normal I was in a better position to stand up for myself.

I had a word with a nurse in the alcove off the main corridor. The nurse was a rebel against the system and was happy to confide in me secrets about the running of the hospital. He and I were good friends and used to go drinking together. I was said by some nurses to have improved but he told me that many still thought that I was ill, that I was just "masking" the symptoms. They were claiming that I had been in the system so long I knew it in and out and that I was well-equipped to dupe the doctors which they said was what I was doing. In fact I was the one who had been duped and was perfectly frank about myself. But they said I was potentially homicidal, that I was hearing voices and seeing things, all a load of nonsense. I should have been acquitted four years previously. I was dismayed and angry at the nurse's words. However pleasant many nurses were on the surface they were deep down just as unenlightened about psychiatric patients as the average man on the street. It did not matter what I said or did, I still found myself in the wrong. Indeed the nurses were inclined to believe the worst about me from reading the malicious psychiatric reports. I now ceased to think of the majority of them as feeling human beings who I could relate to or respect. I was one of the casualties of the system. The nurses observations of me had been wrong as with their deductions and treatment. They didn't remotely understand and never would.

I received a letter on the ward from my father which I eagerly tore open. My father wrote regularly and I appreciated his letters which kept me up to date with the latest information. A new problem had arisen. The doctor in Durban who had previously agreed to have me had left to take up another post in another area without informing his successor about me. This setback had been discovered quite by chance by my father who had then written to Dr. U.. New negotiations had to be opened up with another doctor in South Africa. That hurdle was to take several months to overcome.

At a ward round I entered the office and settled down in a chair opposite Dr. Pears. I mentioned my proposed return to South Africa. She said that the department of health were now unwilling to part with the money for myself and an escort and she said she would write off to them and chase them up on it. I found it difficult to follow the workings of bureaucracy which had a knack for procrastination. I also wondered why I needed an escort. My parents had offered to pay my fare. I was obviously seen not to be trusted to make my own way to South Africa alone. I said to Dr. Pears that I thought the all-round delay might have something to do with the fact that I had been to Broadmoor. She retorted: "You're just paranoid." Paranoid was the word doctors always applied to a person who disagreed with them. My sister and parents who had not been patients in Broadmoor had had no delays in getting to South Africa.

But Dr. Hudson remained a support and he asked me if I would like to be the subject of another case conference, one that he was conducting. Feeling that this might help my case I agreed. The case conference was to be held at the school at Digby and Dr. Hudson drove me there together with a delightful young nurse called Mandy who had not read my case notes and who had asked if she could come along. I had to wait in a classroom; Mandy remained with me in preference to going into the conference. After half an hour I was called in to the sunlit conference room and sat down in a chair next to Dr. Hudson. A whole sea of faces confronted me, nurses, doctors, psychologists. There must have been thirty people in all. In calm encouraging tones Dr. Hudson began with a series of questions on my case and I was later told I answered them very well. Dr. Hudson had already described in graphic detail my prison and Broadmoor experiences together with clinical details of my case. When I was sitting in the lobby at the end of the conference the two nursing tutors from Exe Vale came out and the first turned to me and said: "You've been through a terrible ordeal." I gathered that the whole room wondered why I had been sent to Broadmoor. Dr. Hudson certainly saw life through fresh eyes and with fresh enthusiasm but whatever had been discussed before and during the case conference was to make no difference to my status or how long I remained detained. It was purely of academic interest and was soon forgotten about as I too was forgotten about.

At this time Elizabeth began to probe me as to where I had been for the three years prior to my coming to Exe Vale for I had mentioned that I had been locked up for that length of time. We were talking alone in the waiting room away from listening ears. I hedged and made excuses for my past embarrassed me but Elizabeth was very shrewd and perceptive and she began to suggest I had been to Broadmoor. It emerged that she had once lived in Bracknell which was not far from Broadmoor and she had some knowledge of the place. She also knew Ron who had been to Broadmoor and who was an outpatient at Exe Vale, Wonford. He had overreacted when someone with a knife had attacked him wresting the knife from his attacker and turning it on him ending up with a death on his hands. He was a very imaginative artist and Elizabeth said to me that a reporter from a local newspaper had come to interview him about his paintings. A fabricated story emerged in the next day's paper with the headline Killer Walks Free. The reaction of some people to him in the hospital was of fear and his experience also frightened me off revealing my past to Elizabeth. I held out for sometime but it was difficult when the nurses kept on mentioning Broadmoor in connection with me and eventually I admitted the fact to her.

Elizabeth and I did however cuddle and whisper sweet nothings in each others ears though she would not let me kiss her and this puzzled me. She said: "I could take you seriously if you hadn't been to Broadmoor." I concluded that because I had been to Broadmoor I would always be suspect. Despite all we stuck together.

Shortly after this Elizabeth was discharged and it was then that our understanding deepened. She was in the process of being divorced and she had been obliged to find a bedsit in Exeter. Her new address was 12 Park road, a Victorian terraced house. The walls were dripping with water, there were black patches of damp in the ceiling and at first she had to settle for a kitchen sink and stove in her room. But she was free and I had permission to visit her in her bedsit. It was our first time truly alone together. I lay with her on the bed; we were kissing and cuddling. What ensued was quite natural. It wasn't a brilliant success. In fact it wasn't a success at all. But her tolerance and understanding combined with a deeper understanding of sex on my part meant that on future occasions I was to earn considerable praise. In bed I was dominant but drugs and a programme of psychological terrorism by the state authorities combined with a moral outlook had taken away much vital aggression and only on one occasion did I truly enjoy myself. Afterwards Elizabeth, who was actually a strong woman, behaved like a slave towards me.

I was in a ward meeting with Dr. Pears and Dr. Hudson. Christmas was approaching. Dr. Pears had wagered me a bottle of champagne that I would be back in South Africa by Christmas for my three months would have been long up and she handed over the bottle of champagne, all beautifully corked and coiffured. But though I was still in Exe Vale she said she would get permission from the Home Office for me to go and spend two nights with the Whitakers in Payhembury.

These were to be my first nights away from an institution for over three years. It was lovely to be in the country again with green pastures and cows grazing just a few yards away at   the edge of the garden. My bed was complete with eiderdown and electric blanket and I had my own wardrobe, dressing table and washbasin. When I woke up in the morning it was great not to be bound by a compulsory early morning breakfast but being able just to sink back into a lengthy lie in instead. It was like being truly free again. At the unwrapping of the Christmas presents on Christmas day my family used to be present when we lived in Payhembury. But though they were now out in South Africa there was still the hint of childhood Christmases with the lights on the Christmas tree twinkling and the smiles as we received our presents. I was also able to keep telephone contact with Elizabeth who had gone to her sister's for Christmas along with her young son by her previous marriage.

Though Christmas passed off quite happily, after Christmas Elizabeth suddenly became very cold towards me. Her attitude was not unlike that shown towards a boyfriend she had jilted when she met me. A little before she had been slightly cutting towards me on the ward when a male nurse had sided and abetted with her by trying to make out falsely that I was very dangerous. Although she hadn't shown this side of her nature to me very much she could be nasty and that had led her husband to beat her up several times and her ex-boyfriend to try and throttle her. The point was that she had a dominant bias which I found a challenge and though she liked me subdued it was only a happy relationship when I assumed control. On this occasion I told a nurse to send her away should she visit me at the hospital again.

Unfortunately Dr. Hudson was informed of my fall out with her and I was called into the office where Dr. Hudson and a couple of male nurses were present. I was asked about the breakup, it was a sore subject, and in a moment of weakness a couple of tears formed. Two nurses were amazed that I should display this reaction though I had heard of plenty of dominant males who had displayed such a reaction. And I was surprised that rather than offering a bit of advice and reassurance the response was to cancel all my leave. Prohibition and not "treatment" was as always the order of the day. I felt for a moment that no one had any faith in me and that was the last time I was to mention such a disagreement. I thought that hospitals had nothing to offer and that it as for me to sort out my difficulties myself.

After a week I had forgotten about Elizabeth. Then a blonde-haired girl, pretty though plumpish with a natural timidity that at that time in my eyes made her seem rather dull followed me down the corridor to the kitchen where we filled and switched on the kettle pouring ourselves a cup of tea each. She was wearing a red dress that made her stand out and we got talking. When there is a mutual attraction or a mutual desire to get to know one another the formation of a relationship is the easiest thing in the world. Regrettably she wasn't on my intellectual wavelength.

I was not too disappointed when Elizabeth started to visit the hospital again. At first I tried to send her away as I did not want a resumption of the anguish that a personality like hers could wreak. One day she persuaded me to talk to her and she grabbed my hand and led me round the hospital grounds in the way she used to. It was evening, the sun was sinking over the horizon and long shadows were being cast over the driveway and lawns. Nobody was around and it was very peaceful. Elizabeth was very warm and she told me she loved me. Our separation had allowed her to reappraise her feelings. I told her to think about it and to come back in a week if she still felt inclined. In three days she was back, her feelings unchanged and I started to see her again. I was not strictly allowed out of the hospital grounds and had to play on the good nature of the doctors to regain that little piece of freedom that I had lost. I had had a further test as far as the real world was concerned but having experienced the horror of being locked up indefinitely in Broadmoor I now found the pressures of loving trivial.

About now I was watching the television in the lounge when there was a report about Alan Reeve. He had made a dramatic escape from Broadmoor and had been living in Amsterdam. He was caught in a gun battle with the police killing one and seriously injuring another; he himself was shot and wounded.

One day a curious thing happened that did make me seriously consider my status as a patient on the ward. A female nurse in her early twenties with blond flowing hair and two big eyes bringing into relief her small pretty oval face, became pregnant. She was quite friendly to me and a couple of others and had escorted us down to the pub on a couple of occasions. But then a joke went round that I was the one who had made her pregnant. When she heard about it she was shocked to the core and totally put off. She felt no shame at being pregnant out of wedlock but the notion of a patient being responsible was enough to drive her crazy. She vigorously went out to deny it and I knew that however friendly she had appeared she was only being patronizing and definitely thought of patients as freaks. I saw through the psychiatric reports and labels; I knew that everyone fitted somewhere in the personality spectrum and that it was possible to apply a psychiatric label to anyone, no matter who he was. I just saw a number of patients as having had a raw deal from life and the notion that that made them freaks never entered my mind. That included me. But the nurse was totally lacking in insight, she had swallowed unquestioningly the defamatory reports made on me and however kindly a nurse might treat you now saw clearly that underneath it all too many still regarded us as psychological freaks. My self-confidence naturally remained at a low ebb.

If I did not seek or score any successes with the nurses I was at least not faced with such barriers in my relations with patients. One evening I drank a bottle of wine in my room then staggered in a drunken haze down the corridor to the room of a youngish female patient. My memory of the incident is slightly blurred but poking my head through the door she invited me in. The patient was slim and pretty, her one flaw being her slightly rounded shoulders. She was seated on the bed but out of politeness I sat down on the bare floor. Outside it was dark and in the penumbral gloom only her outline was visible. She started to go on about how love was completely missing from her life. I responded that she had her parents who both loved her but she argued it was not the same thing. She was referring to romantic love. She said how much she loved Dr. Hudson and how much she loved me. Fancied would have been a better word. Then as lithe as a cat she climbed off her bed stripping off her clothes and throwing them onto the floor. White and naked she lay down near me her legs apart. She was dripping but for the first time in my life I had become the victim of brewers droop and I avoided divesting myself of any of my clothes. I had been decidedly short of women trying to seduce me and inevitably the incident stuck in mind.

Some weeks later Dr. Hudson stopped me in the corridor downstairs and said he was leaving Exe Vale. As a parting gesture he said I could go out for six hours a day. He was very flattering about my abilities and said that it would be advisable for me to return to South Africa adding that there would always be disputes as to whether I should have been sent to Broadmoor but the fact remained that I had been sent there and that I could do nothing about it. He continued saying that doctors thought first about themselves and their reputations, not the patient, and that was something I would have to live with. He concluded that I should become something like a farm manager. I concluded that he might be a fledgling psychiatrist but that he had potential to be an eagle in his sphere.

I made a phone call from the telephone booth in the corridor to my parents in South Africa to find out what was happening, a whole load of ten pence pieces stacked on the coin box in front of me. By this means and letter I had gained a picture of events. My mother who was feeling disillusioned had said categorically to my father: "Andrew is not going to come out." My parents had both phoned Dr. U. from South Africa and he had said he was just going to get the go-ahead from the South African Embassy in London. They had just referred the matter to the Department of the Interior in South Africa. My parents had sent my

215

cousin, a lawyer, to the Department of the Interior and he had give them a letter. Though it was supposed to be designed to help me it was just another useless bit of paper. But South Africa's reaction to a reading of the deliberately malicious reports was inevitable. I rang off. Sometime later, at my mother's insistence, my father, who had not been offered a satisfactory job in South Africa, flew back to England and was offered the parish of Marystowe and adjoining parishes in West Devon. Dr. Pears said that if my mother returned to this country as well she would press for my discharge over here.

At this time the psychiatric reports on me were causing a stir amongst the nurses on the ward so after I had complained about them they were removed from the ward. But clearly in such an atmosphere of suspicion and contempt, inevitable from a superficial reading of those dubious documents, it was difficult to maintain a healthy confident attitude. Also the endless ward meetings and regimentation, though perhaps serving some sort of purpose for a newly admitted patient in the acute phase of his illness, were inappropriate for a long stay patient like me. So I asked to be moved to the less stringent regime of Oak.

Oak ward was, as I had hoped, free and easy in comparison to the Bucknill centre. Although the patients were mostly old there were a few of my age whom I got on well with. One had chased a policeman with an axe and had been put on a short term section in an open hospital. Although he was said to suffer from paranoia he was to all intents and purposes quite normal and had just got on the wrong side of the police. He felt that he could get over aggressive and that the drugs calmed him down and though I never saw him behave in a belligerent manner if he felt anti-psychotic drugs were helping him he was entitled to take them though I objected to suppressive drugs being forced on people. Another chap had been abandoned by his wife, he was even denied access to the children and he was very depressed over his situation. He later hung himself in his larder at home. A third patient was depressed and disturbed in other ways and was said to suffer from schizophrenia. His end was not too pleasant either. Oak ward had a side door opening onto a steep fire escape and in the daytime it was customary to leave it open. The drop from the landing was considerable. One day I entered the ward and found the door locked. The patient was nowhere to be seen and I was led to conclude he had jumped. There was also a patient on the ward who had been locked up in Broadmoor for six years. He had seen a chap physically abusing his children and in anger at this grabbed hold of a shotgun and shot him. He had been stricken by remorse, something he was unable to free himself from. He in contrast to most of the murderers I had met, felt he had been treated too leniently saying that there was another patient in Broadmoor who had spent twenty years there for

216

the comparatively minor offence of having sexual intercourse with a cow. The disparity in time it was said led him to shoot himself.

During my time in custody I had plenty of opportunity to view nursing practices and the doctors approach to patients. I remained concerned about the label of madness that I had to wear and totally confused by the methods and theories used to make a diagnosis. One day I happened to glance at the cardex which was lying open on the desk in the charge nurse's office. A female nurse had written of a male patient that his paranoia was still manifesting itself in the fact that he thought people were making derogatory remarks about him behind his back. The patient was an isolated individual unable to begin making friends. I myself knew that people ran him down behind his back. For example on one occasion his lack of success with the opposite sex was brought to ridicule. I also perceived that he gave the appearance of being a little slow and this was why he was a natural target of fun. But so obsessed were the staff (and indeed the doctors) with their theories that they were blind to the reality. And instead of helping the patient he had instead been given a label of madness. Not only was the label wrong it was something he would have to live with for the rest of his life and as I myself knew from experience it could be a prime social handicap. Clearly the "professionals" were quite lacking in true insight and it was no wonder what they had to say did not add up in my mind.

I began to accept my life in Exe Vale. The thing that primarily kept me going was my own inexhaustible capacity for dreaming up schemes for the future, schemes that would allow me to fit back into society and live like a normal human being. All too often ex-Broadmoor patients would find the pressures imposed on them too much leading them to kill themselves or rarely others. I did not let the fact that I had been to Broadmoor weigh on me.

Amongst my schemes for the future was that of getting a good job. I was now also taking an interest in writing hoping some day to get some of my work published. On my bed in my room which I shared with one other patient, I sat with a byro scrawling down my experiences on A.4 paper. At first I found the art of writing difficult but as the cogs of my brain which had been rusted up over time began to turn, thoughts started to flow and gradually my story began to unfold in all its drama. I determined from the start to make my writing a regular thing hoping that in a year I would have completed my memoirs. It was, after a couple of redrafts, to take much longer than that.

In the alcove downstairs I showed a nurse a page of my writing. He slowly perused the page and then he looked up and commented: "Now people would want to read that." He asked me why I was doing it. I replied that I just wanted to get things off my chest. I was also looking for a sense of achievement and just hoped

217

that my book would make sense to anyone who had read my case notes. The nurse looked at things in a more superficial way speculating I was writing for money suggesting I get my story published in the News of the World.

One day I walked into the charge nurse's office when a small ginger-haired patient with thick horn-rimmed spectacles came up to me and put his hands round my throat squeezing tightly and shutting off my oxygen supply. My reaction to an outsider might have seemed strange. I refused to resist right up to the point I found myself passing out. Then I started to struggle involuntarily. It was as if I had made a decision. Fighting back meant violence and I had learned that for some people to fight back was to ask to be locked up. In my case that meant Broadmoor and that was worse than the prospect of death.

No sooner had I broken free than the patient directed a sharp kick at my testicles. As I staggered backwards it never entered my head to retaliate though my anger, slow to manifest itself, was being aroused. Afterwards a male nurse who had witnessed the incident came up to me in the corridor and said:

"Why don't you take him to court?"

My view was sadly more practical. For one thing I regarded litigation as dirty. The stronger party rather than the party with right on its side won and it tended to multiply the suffering and unpleasantness. More significantly I felt as I had done the first day I entered a psychiatric ward that I was somehow no longer taken seriously as a human being. It was as if a mental patient did not enjoy protection under the law, something that the psychiatric and legal professions endorsed by their attitude. A woman patient was strangled to death after being discharged. The girl who killed her was given probation. One reason she didn't get life was that her victim had been in a mental hospital.

At this time Elizabeth became pregnant. It was a happy time and we speculated on the child's sex. Would it be a boy or a girl? We somehow expected it would be a girl and thought of a name, Imogen. But people said having a child was not a wise idea. Would Elizabeth be able to look after it? She was a good mother but was persuaded to have a termination. It was the one thing that caused me guilt. I wish I had been strong enough to prevent it. It is argued that it is cruel to bring a deformed child into the world. I had long since ceased to think of a big percentage of people in psychiatric hospitals as being fundamentally abnormal. Most of their problems were to do with learning and upbringing. The argument that you would be passing on faulty genes I now tended to reject. Afterwards I felt the termination wrong.

My mother was now back in England and my parents were installed in the vicarage at Marystowe. The way was now open for me to be formally interviewed by the psychiatrist for my new catchment area, Dr. Conway. I was at home on short leave and my parents and I drove to the local cottage hospital in Tavistock. My parents were called in first then my turn came. I sat down resolving to be as frank, open and precise as my remaining drugs would permit. They did slow my thinking and muddle my speech. Dr. Conway, a man of friendly appearance and gold-framed spectacles did not approach me with preconceived ideas. I thus felt in no way intimidated and began with determination. I was careful to qualify all my statements and when I spoke of my thought to set the campus ablaze on the day of my arrest I added: "I don't mean with paraffin." Due to the endemic paranoia amongst psychiatrists a figurative turn of phrase could lead to dangerous misinterpretations. I spoke with calmness of peoples savage treatment of me once I had come adrift and I was amazed that he accepted my strongly held belief that people should behave in a moral fashion. I felt I was talking to a genuine physician rather than a prosecutor come judge come jailor. At the end he asked: "Do you feel resentful?" I replied "No" as up till that point I had retained a philosophical attitude. And that concluded the interview.

It was sometime before I was discharged into the fridge of the outside world. In fact it was January 1983. I worked out I had been locked up for four years and ten months. Oscar Wilde spoke of a released prisoner having to crawl to some hole to curl up and die. I still had decades to wait to die but with my reputation in tatters, with little prospect of a job, and without a true male beauty to fall back on anymore, several big question marks still hung over my life. What I had discovered in my journey into the human psyche did disturb, frighten and even revolt me reinforcing my own personal experience. And it was all too clear that what had happened had poisoned many aspects of my life pointing occasionally to the logic of suicide. But I had learned something, I had a torch, the torch of understanding, showing me a way out of the dark night of the soul and illuminating a path into the future.

Note. This volume represents the start of my written journey towards a full understanding of psychiatry and the system and is as relevant now as ever because of what has happened subsequently. I hope and trust that all who read it and who knew me will see that it is a complete, accurate and full account of my first twenty five years. It forms the basis of all the volumes to follow and they are all interdependent. I was to spend three peaceful years under Dr. Conway. Then Mr Fellows, husband of Enid, wrote to say that I had been trapped and framed. I had always maintained that I had been framed but the word trap made me realise I was innocent. At first I had been concerned that I had not been totally in control for those

219

few seconds when trapped but having described it all carefully and in detail no one had the decency to tell me it was a trap as was obvious to anyone looking in on it. But I was to discover that a miscarriage of justice was just the excuse for an orgy of abuse by society and to a significant degree authority. The media were not interested in the truth, the only emphasis all-round was to give me what is called schizophrenia, in effect a spiritual disease and so destroy me, as a psychiatric patient is a valuable source of pain in society and you never surrender a victim. On receiving Mr Fellows letters I suddenly went partially deaf. After a long saga of abuse I was then pressurised to see this homeopathic doctor who gave me ultrasound round the temples to bring down an ear inflammation and I had my pictorial imagination damaged. Although I won my tribunal to lift my life section I was never allowed my freedom and was engaged in a seven year running battle with psychiatry and the system as it threw all it could at me. Eventually what it did to me was the most horrible thing I have ever known happen to anyone. In September 1993, having been hospitalised yet again I stabbed an occupational therapist, something in fact totally out of character, to publicise my pain and ultimately get a Crown Court platform to describe and so hopefully halt the worst persecution I have ever known. But I was just carted off to Broadmoor again with a host of attendant lies. The problem had its origins with what happened to me at university and Mr Fellows, Enid's ex husband, has a dossier of fifteen broken men, the legacy of Enid's thinking though I must say I have not thought of her for very many years. She with the looks and inclination coupled with her experience as a psychiatric nurse, is the most brilliant manipulator I have ever known. I know now that publication is vital to explain myself, society and the system and so bring truth and hopefully some right to bear. With the prospect of the truth coming out I feel the vibes that should restore me though justice depends on my being published.

Lightning Source UK Ltd.
Milton Keynes UK
UKOW052311180712

196238UK00001B/31/A